Get the Real "Skinny" on Healthy Weight Loss

Contrary to What You May have Heard, Weight Loss isn't just about Dieting and Exercise…

It's About Making a Change in your Lifestyle!!!

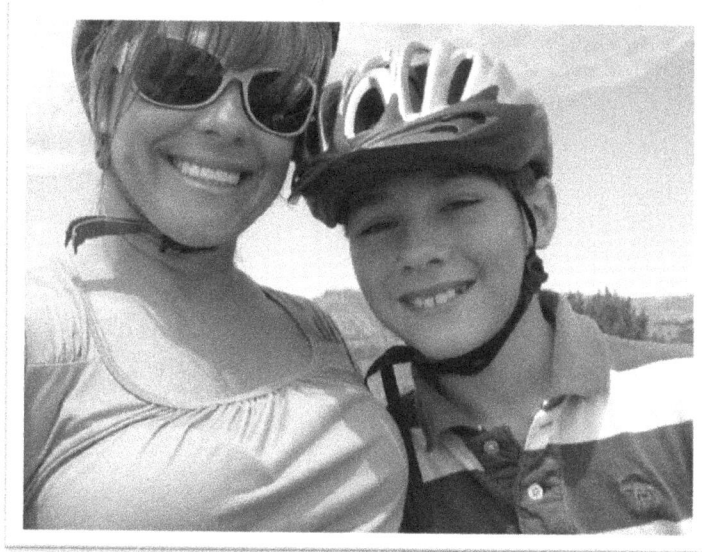

Commit to a Lifestyle Modification and Get Results

Randa Lee Roberts

www.randaleeroberts.com

DISCLAIMER

Any information provided in this guide to healthy weight loss is not intended as medical advice or to replace the medical advice and treatment options provided by your medical physician. As with any weight loss and/or exercise program, all readers are advised to consult with their own doctors and/or health professionals for information pertaining to medical conditions. The author shall be held harmless and is not responsible for misinterpretation of the data contained herein or for any loss, damage or injury allegedly resulting or caused directly or indirectly by any treatment, action or application of any food or food source outlined within this guide. The statements in this book have not been evaluated by the U.S. Food and Drug Administration. Any and all information provided is not intended to diagnose, treat, cure or prevent any form of disease.

Email: Send questions to: surfingturtlebooks@gmail.com
Website: www.randaleeroberts.com

DEDICATION

This guide is dedicated to my father, Joseph Gordon Roberts, who struggled with his weight, high blood pressure, and Type-II diabetes until he lost his battle and was taken from us prematurely. It was due to my constant desire to encourage him to change his "lifestyle" that I was able to learn the many elements necessary to create and sustain a healthy life.

I dedicate this book to anyone who desires to make a positive change in their lives by committing to and implementing the changes that it takes to modify lifelong habits and to bring about the lifestyle changes that they aspire to achieve.

PREFACE

With all of the books about dieting that are found on the market and online these days, you might be asking yourself, "Why do I need more diet information?" Well, the truth is, you probably don't, but how do you really know?

I suppose you could ask yourself a few questions to help determine whether another guide is needed. Do you answer "no" to any of the following questions?

- "Have I been successful at losing weight?"

- "Has my weight loss been more than just water weight?"

- "Am I starving myself or going without items that I enjoy?"

- "Am I taking supplements or harmful weight loss stimulants to lose the weight?"

- "Have I been successful at keeping the weight off – for more than one month? Three Months? Six Months? One year?"

- "Am I within the healthy weight limits as described by my personal physician?"

- "Am I happy? Or am I constantly irritable?"

- "Do I look and feel better about myself?"

If you responded in ways that have made you question your weight loss success, you may need to review the methods with which you've chosen to lose the weight.

Each and every individual that promotes diet, exercise, and weight loss come from different places, usually providing specific information related to their own personal set of circumstances and beliefs. They may be coming from a different place entirely than you. Does this mean that the information provided is irrelevant or completely off base? Absolutely not! It just means that you'll have to read through the information, find specifics to weight loss and exercise that are universal in nature, and apply them to your own situation, which is somewhat predetermined by your lifestyle.

Within the covers of this guide, my goal is to provide you with information that will help you commit to a total lifestyle change, as truly healthy weight loss IS dependent upon every choice that you make and action you take. It's not just about how much you eat or whether you exercise regularly, there are many other factors that come into play. How do I know? I'll share my personal experiences with you later; however, suffice it to say that I've endured a tremendous number of life-changing experiences, each of which has led to this publication.

My beliefs about healthy weight loss may differ from your own, but I promise you they are based on solid research and life experiences, and have been carefully scrutinized and implemented to ensure that they work when applied to every aspect of your life.

TABLE OF CONTENTS

PART ONE

Here and Now

CHAPTER ONE
INTRODUCTION

Thanks for choosing this guide out of all the others available to you. Evidently, you've recognized the need or have a desire to make a commitment to a total lifestyle change. Perhaps you're overweight, or fear that you've made choices in your life that will eventually take their toll on you and your overall health. Maybe you're concerned about a friend or loved one that you see walking down the wrong path. Whatever your reason for making the investment, I hope that you're ready to commit to making the necessary changes in your life so that you can benefit for a lifetime.

Many diet solutions or programs that have provided temporary success to those who've engaged have failed to address the total package, which is the overall lifestyle of the individual seeking a permanent change. For instance, some programs are heavily focused on exercise with little emphasis on healthy eating habits, while others are consumed with caloric intake yet provide few details about proper exercise techniques. In order to see permanent changes in one's health and wellness, all aspects of his/her lifestyle must be changed. That is the focus of this manual.

Get the Real "Skinny" on Healthy Weight Loss is for individuals who've tried the "quick" weight loss programs with little or no lasting success; it's for those who've bought into the pre-packaged "meal" programs as a solution for permanent weight loss at a very hefty price; and for the individual who's tried everything else and still hasn't found the permanent solution that they've been seeking. In other words, it's for everyone. A new way of thinking, eating, exercising, and living.

Are you ready to make the total commitment to change your lifestyle?

Now that I've shared with you the underlying goal of this book, let me share with you the reason I've elected to put it all together for you. Perhaps like you, I woke up one day, looked in the mirror and asked myself, "Who is this person looking back at me?" "Surely this isn't the athletic, physically fit person that once existed in a petite little body, or is it?" Unfortunately it was – and it had to change.

Perhaps, unlike you, I understood the importance of an overall lifestyle change, as I'd lived that life before - before college, marriage, family, career, and the stresses that seem to accompany each element of my existence. So what happened? I got lazy. Yes, I still practiced the basics, but not consistently, and consistency is the key. Without it, you may as well accept who and what you look like now because it will otherwise never change.

I was determined to master my metabolism, which had evidently changed somewhere along the way, and practice my former eating and food preparation techniques while incorporating exercise routines and habits that were more conducive to my age and overall fitness goals. Since I was generating this "Lifestyle" program for myself, it only made sense to put it together for others to use as well.

Modifying your lifestyle will not be easy – but it will be well worth it. If you just keep in mind your final goal, how this information and strategies will lead to positive changes that you'll enjoy and benefit from throughout the course of your lifetime, and remember that this isn't a typical diet in which you have to pass on your favorite foods, just modify the way that you enjoy them, you'll do remarkably well.

Let's make your goal a reality this time around. By following the steps that I've outlined for you in this guide, and really sticking to them, you'll be able to see positive results and achieve success. So let's get started. Are you with me?

CHAPTER TWO
YOUR PERSONAL JOURNAL

In order to achieve success when making a commitment to change your lifestyle, you must first take a close look at your starting point. This can be accomplished in many ways, but I found it easiest to reflect upon photographs of my younger years that I found in a photo album to see where I once was, so that I could then compare images of me from the past to my present.

Although this can be somewhat disheartening, it provides the clearest picture of reality, especially if you've gained weight over the years or allowed yourself to simply get out of shape. So, why put yourself through this torture? I'll tell you why… a picture is worth a thousand words and seeing IS believing!

Once you review and compare where you were to where you are, you'll be able to internalize the changes that need to be made in order to achieve the weight loss that you desire. This provides a pretty strong basis for you to establish your commitment.

If available, I'd like you to attach a "BEFORE" photo of yourself that you like below and then include a photograph of you now. This will be used for your affirmation of change that we'll be using throughout this guide.

BEFORE:

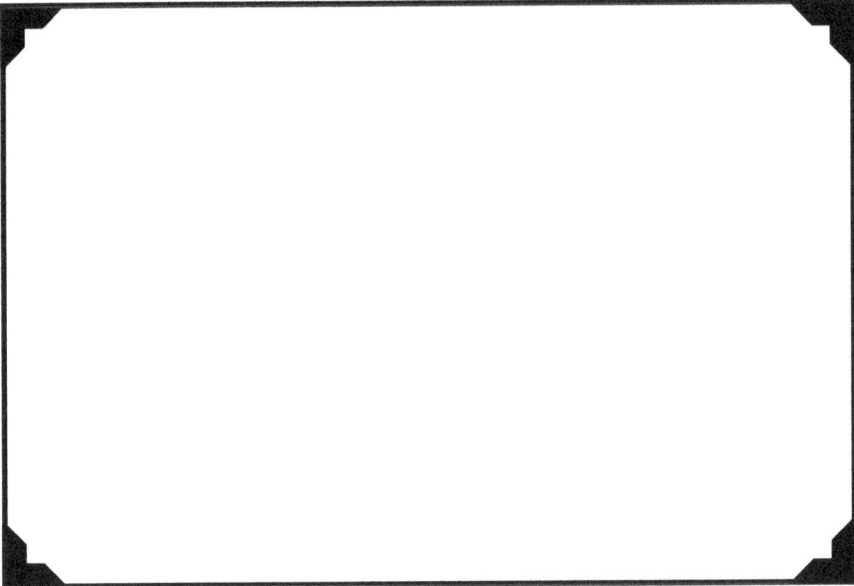

This image was taken in or around the time I was _____ years of age.

NOW:

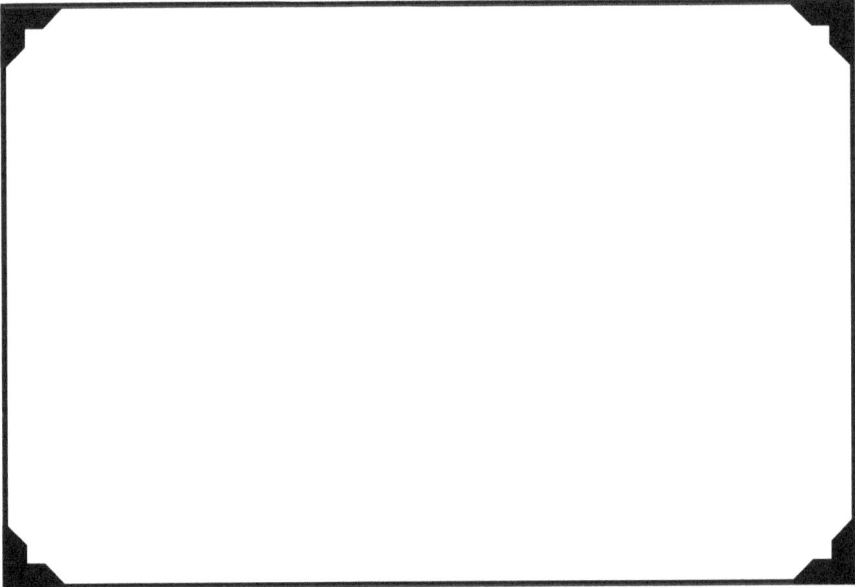

This is a photograph of me now, taken _____.

What is your "Why?"

I know the first step was a difficult one. Having to look at and accept the changes that have occurred during the course of one's lifetime isn't always easy. In fact, it can be quite painful. For me it was absolutely excruciating. Since I could remember, I'd always been fit and trim. I'd been involved in dance as a ballerina; a gymnast; long-distance runner; and a cheerleader; beginning somewhere around the age of three, and I'd never had to worry about my weight.

Guess what? Life changed... I grew up, got married, had a family, and gained weight. I no longer had the "pep in my step" that I'd grown accustomed to enjoying every day. I began to feel aches and pains throughout my body, and became winded when I went on hikes or bike rides.

I wasn't able to keep up with my two athletic boys, and that was when it hit me. I wasn't able to be the mom that I wanted to be. I wasn't able to enjoy the things in life that I should've been enjoying with my children and husband. I was limited and THAT wasn't acceptable. I had to make a change and that is my "why." What's yours?

Make a List of Your "Why(s)":

1)_____

2)_____

3)_____

4)_____

What Have You Done in the Past?

If you're like most people who've struggled with weight loss and dieting, you've probably attempted various exercise and weight loss programs without achieving long-lasting results. I know I have.

As I mentioned before, I'd never struggled to lose weight when I was younger, as I was incredibly active and apparently had a pretty "fast" metabolism, so whatever I ate never stuck around on my thighs, waistline, hips, or love-handles.

Today, however, it's a different story. In my quest to lose weight, I tried counting calories; limiting the types of foods that I consumed according to metabolic typing; I ate multiple "small" meals a day; and joined a gym complete with a personal trainer. I worked with my trainer twice weekly for one hour over the course of four years.

Interestingly enough, I ended my weight training weighing exactly the same as I did when I'd started four years earlier. I was firmer, but I still had the same layer of fat spread over my body. In fact, instead of getting smaller, I appeared to be getting larger – at least that's the story that my clothes told me. I became quite concerned and wondered why nothing was working. I started my research and found that I was doing things incredibly wrong.

What have you tried?

1)_____

2)_____

3)_____

Were Your Efforts Successful or Not?

After working out for four years and growing larger instead of smaller, I knew that the things that I'd been doing were evidently NOT working for me. I was actually eating too few calories. Who knew that was even possible?

I was eating smaller meals throughout the day, but I was still hungry and NOT consuming the number of calories my body needed to thrive. I was forcing my body into starvation mode. This meant that instead of burning calories, my body was holding onto them as reserves. On top of that, my weight training program resulted in lots of muscle mass or bulk and did not reduce or burn fat calories quickly enough, so I actually appeared larger than I looked when I began the program.

Although I was strong as an ox and could lift or do anything for myself, I wasn't the petite individual I desired to be. Hopefully, your results were different than mine. But just in case, let's record them as a baseline for what worked and what did not.

What Were Your Results?

1)_____

2)_____

3)_____

How Would You Describe Yourself Today?

After reading, researching, and learning everything that I could about healthy weight loss and incorporating all of the information into my lifestyle, including better ways to prepare the foods that I provided me and my family, better exercise routines and much, much more, I've been able to lose the weight, firm and tone my body, fit into my clothes (which I refused to get rid of), and I feel great.

I sleep better, my skin has a youthful glow, and my hair and nails are strong and healthy too. In fact, although I'm fiftyish, many individuals with whom I've come into contact think I'm in my thirties. Now that's something to be excited about.

This can be your story too.

How Would You Describe Yourself?

1)_____

2)_____

3)_____

Where do you want to see yourself in three months, six months, one year?

Like many people, I wanted to look like I did in my younger days – 120 pounds soaking wet; a firm, shapely butt and long lean thighs; beautiful calves; sculpted abdominals; a trim back, arms and shoulders; no flab; natural golden brown hair; and the stamina of a racehorse (remember, I was a cross-country runner).

Although some of this was attainable, not all of my desires were realistic. Too many factors had changed: my body's shape, my skin's elasticity or capacity for it, and more. I had to recognize that some areas would never be able to resume their original shape, texture, tone, or functionality.

For instance, after giving birth to my two sons in my thirties, my skin wasn't as supple as it was when compared to my twenties, leaving me with skin that just wouldn't firm up the way I desired it to be. As I aged, my lean legs began to show signs of cellulite, which was nature's way of telling me that I wasn't producing as much collagen, which resulted in a loss of elasticity in my skin, allowing little bumps and dimples to peek through.

And finally, my once-beautiful olive skin was beginning to reflect little spots, remnants of too much sun exposure in my younger years. Once I realized and came to terms with the things that I couldn't change, I painted an image of what I could resolve and focused on changing those areas so that I wouldn't be disappointed in the end. This is important for anyone who desires to make changes to understand. Work toward changing the areas of your life and body that you can modify, and learn to love and accept the things that you cannot change.

Setting realistic goals and expectations is necessary if you truly intend to attain them. Start small and increase them as you begin to see changes. Remember, your goals may include dietary changes or modifications; exercise goals and routines; and physical, emotional and social changes too.

Where do you see yourself in three months?

_____

_____

Where do you see yourself in six months?

_____

_____

Where do you see yourself in one year?

_____

_____

Take Note of the Details:

<u>Before:</u>

Height _____ Date _____

Weight _____ Date _____

Waist _____ Date _____

Buttocks _____ Date _____

Hips _____ Date _____

Thigh _____ Date _____
(Circumference- 10" above knee)

Knee _____ Date _____
(Circumference)

Shoulders _____ Date _____
(Circumference)

Ribcage _____ Date _____
(Halfway between naval & sternum)

Bicep _____ Date _____
(At largest part)

Calve _____ Date _____
(Circumference – 5" below knee)

Ankle _____ Date _____
(At widest part)

Neck _____ Date _____

Pant Size _____ Date _____

Dress Size _____ Date _____

<u>After:</u>

Height _____ Date _____

Weight _____ Date _____

Waist _____ Date _____

Buttocks _____ Date _____

Hips _____ Date _____

Thigh _____ Date _____
(Circumference- 10" above knee)

Knee _____ Date _____
(Circumference)

Shoulders _____ Date _____
(Circumference)

Ribcage _____ Date _____
(Halfway between naval & sternum)

Bicep _____ Date _____
(At largest part)

Calve _____ Date _____
(Circumference – 5" below knee)

Ankle _____ Date _____
(At widest part)

Neck _____ Date _____

Pant Size _____ Date _____

Dress Size _____ Date _____

CHAPTER THREE
YOUR JOURNEY STARTS HERE

A Clean Slate!

Before you start anything, you must rid yourself of any preconceived notions, or perhaps explained another way, a self-fulfilling prophecy. For instance, you cannot pledge to change your lifestyle if you're still holding firmly onto failed past experiences. Moving forward means leaving the past behind you. This is true in many of life's areas.

A failed marriage shouldn't deter you from ever finding happiness again. The loss of a child shouldn't preclude you from having another baby one day. Being terminated from your job wouldn't result in your throwing up your hands and announcing that you'll never work again because you were once let go, would it? I should hope not!

Therefore, none of your previous weight-loss interventions and programs that proved ineffective should prevent you from trying again. Remember the saying, "If at first you don't succeed, try, try again."

So, take a deep breath and repeat after me –

"I can do anything that I set my mind to do;"

"I am a strong, confident, beautiful individual;"

"I am devoted to making the necessary changes in my life to achieve both the physical and emotional goals that I've established for myself!"

Power of Positive Thinking:

Throughout my life's journey, I've maintained a positive attitude, as I learned firsthand and early on that a positive attitude equals a positive outcome. I firmly believe that having a positive outlook in life will make life's journey a much more positive experience as well.

In fact, I can share with you at least one specific incident in which I waivered in my attitude and didn't achieve the desired outcome. While attending college I decided to try out for cheerleading. I was very excited, certainly qualified, but something in the back of my mind made me question my capabilities and myself.

Short version of the story, I didn't make the squad. I doubted myself and it reflected in my attitude and performance. This experience made me realize that as long as I keep positive thoughts flowing, I'll be able to master, accomplish, or achieve any goal I establish for myself. Through the power of positive thought there is very little that one cannot achieve.

I'd like to share a few quotes about positive thinking so that you can share in their powerful influences in your life, and more specifically modifying your lifestyle, in order to achieve the desired healthy weight loss that you're looking to achieve.

- *Positive thinking is expecting, talking, and visualizing with certainty what you want to achieve, as an accomplished fact.*

- *Affirm the positive, visualize the positive, and expect the positive, and your life will change accordingly.*

- *Positive and negative are directions. Which direction do you choose?*

By repeating these phrases each and every day, you'll eventually begin to internalize the underlying messages that are reflected through the words.

Developing a Plan of Action:

Obviously, with any venture that you elect to engage, establishing goals is necessary. Without goals, you're pretty much spinning your wheels and going nowhere. For instance, individuals who are involved in sales will always establish a sales goal that they will work to achieve; gymnasts will decide upon a "stunt" and then establish a deadline and work excruciatingly long hours in order to master it; and students will often decide upon a grade point average that they desire to earn in order to gain admittance to a specific college or university.

Goals are necessary, as is a plan of action, as goals cannot be achieved without a plan. The same philosophy is necessary when implementing a weight loss plan. You may have set a goal to lose a certain amount of weight, but without a specific plan you may not be able to accomplish that weight loss goal. A plan of action is needed and easily accomplished if you know how to approach it.

Having shared that, one of the things that I've found to assist me in establishing and working toward my goals is a calendar. I choose to use an At-A-Glance calendar, which includes quarter-hours so that I can schedule my entire day – this includes the time(s) I'm going to exercise and what exercises I'll be engaging in so that I can maintain a well-balanced program; deadlines which include miscellaneous activities related to my overall desired lifestyle changes; and menus for meals throughout the week so that I can ensure that everything is balanced. Although this may seem tedious, it provides me an outline so that I can easily achieve my goals.

Remember, a goal is only a goal unless you have a plan of action to help you reach and achieve it.

Establishing a Support System:

For athletes who are involved in sports, hearing the cheering fans from the sidelines provides them an extra motivation to succeed. Your goals are no different in the overall scheme of things. Everyone needs someone to lean on, especially when what it is they are trying to accomplish may prove difficult along the way.

Finding someone to share the details of your plan, or perhaps join you in your lifestyle modification, is something that will inspire, motivate, and keep you on track. Having another who will pull you along when you're lagging, or who you can encourage should they fall behind, is an excellent method of ensuring your success.

If you're not married, include a good friend or other relative who loves and cares about you, and who will help you reach your goal and will be available to support you along the way. If you are married, and have a family, your goal will affect everyone within your household. A lifestyle modification will clearly impact the healthy eating habits of those residing under the same roof, which will ultimately affect them too.

By bringing them on board and explaining how the changes that you intend to implement will include changes to their lives too, you'll have not just a support team, but individuals who are just as eager to make positive changes in their lives as well, and who will increase your chances of following through astronomically.

Affirmations & Accountability:

"I know I can," "I know I can" is a positive affirmation that will help you to achieve your desired goals. By telling yourself that you can do something vs. doubting yourself, you'll definitely enjoy more success. Positive thoughts, or through the development of a self-fulfilling prophecy, you'll be able to imagine the outcome of your desired goal and changes that you've decided to change in your life.

For instance, one of my desires was to return home to my thirtieth class reunion and resemble the fit and trim young girl from years before. Positive affirmations made this possible, as I was able to inspire, motivate, and encourage myself each and every day until I achieved this portion of my lifestyle modification. Obviously, this goal required that I make many changes in my lifestyle in order to attain it.

As any parent knows, accountability is the key if you want a child to truly understand how his/her choices impact the end results. For instance, the child that desires to have friends over to visit on Saturday will certainly understand that if he/she does not clean their bedroom or the necessary living space as directed, then he/she will NOT be having friends over to visit.

Making a commitment to change one's lifestyle and then NOT following through will lead to similar end results. If you "fall off the wagon" and stop eating the foods that you know are recommended for losing the unwanted weight that your body holds onto, you'll not lose the weight. If you choose to sit in front of the television eating a bag of chips instead of exercising, you'll more than likely not develop the lean, trim muscles that you desire in order to wear the itty, bitty, bikini on your upcoming cruise.

Everyone can make excuses and everyone will waiver from time to time, but holding oneself accountable for their choices will make a difference. For instance, establishing consequences for your "lack of willpower" will certainly make you think twice about eating four scoops of ice cream before bed. How? Well, suppose one of your short-term goals is to go on a cruise in three months IF, and only if, you're able to wear your previous wardrobe, including shirts, shorts, swimwear, and evening wear. If you don't achieve your goal, you don't go on the cruise. Plain and simple!

CHAPTER FOUR
FACTORS INFLUENCING OR SABOTAGING YOUR HEALTHY WEIGHT GOALS

You may not believe this, but there may be outside influences that could affect your ability or perhaps your journey to reach your goals. Recognizing these outside factors and/or influences ahead of time will be the key to your success. Remember, most goals are attainable, although you may experience an obstacle or two along the way. Being aware of these specific factors will help you adjust your plan of action so that they will NOT deter your eventual success.

Taking a look at predetermined factors such as your age, the environment that you have to work within, your personal genetics, and your capacity for change are all things you'll want to consider, as obviously, some of these factors cannot be modified. Finding a healthy, happy compromise that you can live with will be necessary in order for your overall goals to be reached. Let's take a look at these factors and how they'll make a difference in your plans for lifestyle modification.

Age Plays a Role:

As none of us want to readily admit it, our age plays a tremendous role in the things that we do and elect NOT to do. It is also a factor that controls many of our body's internal functions, which ultimately impact what happens on the outside. For instance, when I was fifteen years of age, I wouldn't hesitate to climb the tallest tree along the back of our property.

It was excellent for strengthening my upper body to complement my lower body strength and muscle mass that I'd developed through cross-country running, and it provided me an incredible opportunity to see things far off in the distance while it increased my capacity for reacting calmly when faced with scary or intense situations (like breaking tree limbs or the occasional snake resting on a branch). Today, unless I had to rescue a child or one of our cats, I'd pass on the tree climbing adventure.

Why? First of all, let's just say that I'm not nearly as adventurous (or perhaps haphazard, or stupid) as I once was. Secondly, what's the point of climbing to the top of a tree to see when my eyes aren't nearly as strong and capable as they were when I was fifteen? Last of all, I've had two babies naturally, so I'm about as calm and brave as a woman can be when experiencing frightening or "tense" situations.

Age will prevent individuals from doing things that they'd truly like to do. I'm pretty sure that most fifty-five-year-old men aren't going to strap on some equipment and play football with boys one-fourth their age, just as I'm not going to attempt a backflip on the trampoline anytime soon. I think you get the point. With age, unfortunately, comes certain limitations to our abilities and what we consider necessary to attain our goals.

Metabolism:

Part of the "age" thing mentioned above are changes that occur within our bodies. One of the most noticeable changes that we have to deal with is that of our metabolism. Yes, it's a fact, as we get older our metabolism slows down... to some of us it appears to have come to a complete halt.

Where we were once able to eat anything that our hearts desired without worrying or repeating the age-old saying, "A minute on the lips, a lifetime on the hips," I now ask myself, "Is it worth it?" Usually the answer is yes, which is why a lifestyle modification is the way to go about healthy weight loss. You don't have to give up all of the good stuff in life – you just have to be smarter about how you go about enjoying them.

Genetics:

Now, for the most part, we'd all like to be the sexy vixen at the beach sporting the string bikini that the men just can't get enough of. In fact, my husband's eyes have had to be retrieved several times, as they've literally popped out of his head and rolled along the pavement or landed in the sand. Bad husband... bad! Maybe you're one of those individuals who only need to look at the treadmill and immediately notice a difference in your physical appearance. Maybe you're not!

Genetics play a major role in our physical appearance, from the color of our hair, eyes, and skin tone to the shape of our bodies along the way. Although not every aspect of our appearance and/or existence is dictated by genetics, plenty of them will be. For instance, I'm Italian from my mother's side of the family, and what we'll refer to as Heinz 57 on my dad's side. Pretty much a crapshoot as to how I would turn out as I grew and matured.

As a child my hair took on my father's shade – sandy blonde. I was blessed with the capacity for tanning easily, as my skin tone was "olive" and provided from my mother. My father was 5 feet 10 inches and my mother was 4 feet 9 inches. Luckily for me, genetics split the difference and I'm 5 feet 4 inches.

Sure, I'd love to have an extra couple of inches, but that's why high heels were invented. My mother has dark brown eyes and my father had beautiful blue eyes – I was born with hazel eyes with more blue tones than brown. You see my point here? We have to work with what we are provided at birth. You can't change everything (unless you have an excellent plastic surgeon) and/or just because you want too. You can, however, tweak what you already have.

Body Type(s):

This section is for individuals who, no matter what they've tried, just cannot change the shape of their body or have noticed a particular pattern taking place regarding their shape. Believed by Holistic Health and Weight Loss experts to play a significant role in our body's overall shape, I found that there truly is a parallel, and you may too.

In order for this to make sense, you need to understand that within your body you have three fat-storing hormones and six fat-burning hormones. It's also important to understand that diet and exercise alone will NOT burn fat, but instead will stimulate the glands in your body to create fat-burning hormones. Sounds great so far – right? Not quite. Why? Because if your glands are weak or damaged, your body will not produce enough of the fat-burning hormones needed to burn the fat. When this happens, your body will begin to store fat around the weakened or damaged glands within your body and your shape will begin to change. You may even begin to develop symptoms.

It is at this point that individuals need to understand that a "one size fits all" mentality will not work when it comes to weight loss and exercise. For instance, if your adrenal glands are weak or damaged, they aren't doing their job. The wrong kind of exercises can actually result in weight gain instead of weight loss. It's good to know if you have a specific deficiency so that your plan of action can take this into account.

To make your weight loss goals realistic, let me identify a few "Body Types" that will help you to understand if your weight gain or failure to lose can be attributed to any of the deficiencies listed below.

Adrenal Body Type

First of all, let me describe where the adrenals are located and what they do. The adrenal glands can be found right above your kidneys. Their job is to produce adrenal hormones, which are responsible for controlling your sleep and wake cycles. If you suffer from adrenal problems, it seems that your sleep/wake cycles are backwards. Typically you're tired during the day even though you are usually unable to sleep through the night.

During the evening when you're supposed to be resting peacefully, you simply cannot relax enough to fall into the deeper sleep cycles that your body requires. As a result, you'll often feel fatigued; are frequently the victim or excessive stress, worry, anxiety and depression; and suffer from brain fog or dullness. You simply aren't yourself.

If you suffer from adrenal exhaustion, you'll more than likely observe excessive fat storage or weight in and around the midsection. You may find it difficult to fit into your clothing. Some people will resort to girdles or elastic bands to help hold the "belly fat" in, but this is dangerous, as these bands can actually constrict vital organs within the abdomen. You may notice puffiness around your face and eyes, a double chin, and a rounding of the face. Dark circles around and/or beneath the eyes isn't uncommon and may result in an overall "tired" appearance.

Thyroid Body Type

This is the body type that I hear most people complain about when they're discussing their inability to lose weight. When the thyroid gland is the culprit, it usually requires a specialized dietary and exercise program. It is always best to visit your doctor to allow him/her to create a program that will best suit your needs. In addition, he/she may prescribe dietary supplements or prescription medications, which will support and improve your thyroid function.

Individuals suffering from thyroid issues will often notice loose or sagging skin under the arms, chin or midsection due to body proteins responsible for keeping the skin firm breaking down faster than it can replenish itself. People who suffer with thyroid issues will often have cold hands and/or feet, resulting in a need to wear socks to bed at night to keep them warm, and often extra clothing to feel comfortable even in moderate climates.

When one suffers with thyroid issues, it isn't uncommon for them to crave sugary carbohydrates like pasta, cereals, crackers, pancakes, waffles, donuts, cakes, muffins, rice cakes, cookies, candy, chocolate, juice, alcohol, wine, beer, ice cream and breads. This is because everything within the body is slower and the body desires quick energy resulting from carbohydrates.

There are a few identifiable symptoms that individuals who have a thyroid body type may possess, like vertical ridges on their nails; hair falling out; and excessive weight gain all over.

Ovary Body Type

When the ovaries aren't functioning properly, the result is an imbalance of progesterone and estrogen, which may cause more fat. This fat is then stored on the body in areas such as "saddlebags," thighs, and the lower stomach and buttocks. In the lower abdomen, it will be stored just below the bellybutton as an unsightly bulge.

Typical problems of the ovaries may include PMS (premenstrual syndrome); cravings and/or bloating at certain times of the month; extra painful cramping; depression during the menstrual cycle; "HOT" flashes; and excessive bleeding.

Liver Body Type

Last of all are problems related to an improperly functioning liver. Often individuals who have a weakened or challenged liver will put on excessive weight around the abdomen. Bodily aches and pains are not unusual and will often feel like a tight, arthritic-like feeling in the lower back, especially in the mornings. Fingers and joints can also become swollen.

Many individuals who suffer from a poorly functioning liver will often complain of tightness or pain in the right shoulder or right side of the neck. Many times they'll swear it is an old injury, but after exhaustive treatments, the pain never dissipates long term. Individuals will often find it difficult to awaken in the morning and frequently complain about a heavy and/or dull ache in the forehead and neck area.

Recognizing that sometimes there are physical ailments that are contributing to your weight loss and/or gain is critical to understanding what you should be doing to "heal" the gland associated with the storage of fat on your body.

Seeking medical care and assistance is always the best course of action if you feel that something is responsible for your physical appearance. If you prefer to seek assistance from your primary medical practitioner, I'd recommend that you do so. If not, there are other resources available, such as alternative care practitioners.

Disease, Disability and Disposition:

This particular segment is a tough one but one, nonetheless, that we need to address. Obviously, some diseases are genetically passed from one generation to another, and perhaps your lifestyle modification will have to include special treatments, meals, medications, etc., as a result.

Maybe you were injured during the course of your lifetime, leaving you without the full use of your body; or perhaps you suffer from illnesses that preclude you from doing things that you desire to do, enjoy, and/or participate in.

The beauty of a lifestyle modification is that you get to decide what you do, how you do it, if it's practical, convenient and/or realistic. Nobody else gets to determine it for you (unless you have to include the advice of your medical practitioner, which is obviously in your best interest as he/she will know your physical, emotional, and social limitations). Your doctor may actually be available to assist you in determining a workable plan and solution to help you achieve your goals.

PART TWO

Understanding the Facts that Make the Difference

CHAPTER FIVE
CALORIE COUNTING VS. HEALTHY EATING HABITS

Do you know what the single most important or exciting part about a lifestyle makeover is? It is the fact that you get to make changes to everything that you feel is necessary in your life to help you achieve your ultimate goals of healthy weight loss and a healthier, happier you. It's a free "Do-Over."

The opportunity for you to evaluate your lifestyle, habits, complete with challenges that you must contend with, and then "fix them" to provide you a chance to do it all over again, making better choices or decisions so that you can achieve and enjoy total happiness. What an incredible opportunity. You might be asking yourself, "How am I going to do that?" Well, I'm about to show you. This is the "Good" part!

Calorie – Friend or Foe?

All right, I know that I told you there would be no more calorie counting, but I feel the need to educate you about what a calorie actually is. So, without further ado, let's tackle the "calorie."

According to Webster's Dictionary, a calorie is for measuring the energy produced by food when oxidized in the body;

A calorie, as defined by medical dictionary, http://www.thefreedictionary.com/, now used only in metabolic studies, is used to express the fuel or energy value of food. It is equivalent to the kilocalorie.

Truly, however, a calorie is actually a unit of heat energy. More specifically, one calorie is the amount of energy needed to increase the temperature of one gram of water by one degree centigrade.

Calories from food are needed in order for your body to function properly. For instance, your body will "burn" calories to breathe, digest food, maintain organs and their systems, as well as to lose weight. If a body doesn't receive enough calories, then it will begin breaking down muscle mass in order to function properly. This is not limited to muscles that you might find in your abdomen, leg, or arm.

The body doesn't care what muscle(s) it absorbs or burns if it can derive the energy needed, which is why a low-calorie diet can actually be harmful. The heart, obviously one of the main muscles within the body, can actually be used for energy if the body decides to use this particular muscle for energy. You and I both know, even without a medical degree, that this cannot be good. In fact, it can be quite dangerous, leading to cardiac atrophy.

Put Away the Calculator:

Yes, that's right. Put away the calculator as you WON'T be counting calories anymore. Healthy weight loss isn't just about calories, counting portions, weighing the foods you eat, etc., although I will include a few caloric charts for your reference. It's about so much more. In fact, it's more about your body and how it processes the foods that you eat.

Each and every person has a unique biochemistry, which means that no two people alive require the same serving sizes or types of foods. Although it's true that everyone needs a balanced diet, finding the correct balance is the key to healthy weight loss. Everyone requires healthy proteins, carbohydrates, and healthy fats in order for their bodies to be properly nourished and able to function its best. But what this means is that there is no "magic" weight loss plan that will work the same way for any two people, which is why it is necessary and to your advantage to learn about your very unique and specific metabolic type. By discovering your metabolic type, you'll be able to establish a customized diet plan, which will provide you with long-term weight loss results that are healthy and a plan that won't leave you feeling hungry all of the time.

Metabolic typing has been around for quite some time, with a lot of information available for individuals who know that this type of information will make all the difference in their weight loss program, and how effective it will be. But, not everyone knows just how important these details can be in losing weight. So, in an effort to keep the details short, sweet, and simple, I'm going to provide you a short lesson in Metabolic Typing.

Every individual in the United States has a Social Security number, which is unique to that person for identifying him or her throughout their lifetime. Well, in much the same way, everyone has a unique Protein Metabolic Type, Carbohydrate Metabolic Type, or Mixed Metabolism Type. So what are they? Let's find out.

Protein Metabolic Types:

- Protein Types – If you are a Protein type, you're an individual who frequently desires foods that aren't necessarily considered to be "healthy" foods. These foods may include those commonly known to be rich and fatty, such as lasagna, bacon, pizza, sausage, and salty nuts. Most people who fall into this category L-O-V-E to eat and will often still feel hungry after eating a large meal. People in this group who've eaten lots of carbohydrates may have cravings for sugar. Often, individuals in this category will desire sugar and typically cannot stop consuming it. And unfortunately, they'll experience the jitters similar to that of a caffeine junky and may even have a sudden loss of energy. People who find themselves in this category may have experienced failed diets in the past, as they attempted calorie-cutting methods that were ineffective. They may have even consumed the wrong types of foods, which caused them to feel a loss of energy. Finally, and most noticeably, individuals in this category suffer from symptoms of fatigue or may feel like they're on the edge. Cycles which include extreme energy ups and downs are typical of a contradiction between metabolic type and food consumption.

What do individuals who've discovered that they are Protein Types need in order to be successful at weight loss?

- Protein types need to eat a diet rich in proteins (45%) and healthy fats (10%) and avoid consuming excessive carbohydrates (35%), as clearly we see what can happen as outlined above. But this doesn't mean that they cannot consume carbohydrates at all. It's more about "balance" and making certain that you keep your diet level. I'm a Libra, which means that I seek balance in all aspects of my life, and that includes my menu. Eating various carbohydrates, such as healthy grains, fruits, and vegetables along with proteins and fats will prove beneficial in your diet and quest to lose weight.

Protein types are able to break down (metabolize) their food more quickly than the other groups, and that means that they often feel a tinge of hunger all of the time if they eat foods low in fat. Eating heavier proteins such as eggs (instead of just the whites), red meats, dairy, and poultry (especially the dark meat) are essential to their dietary needs and will often eliminate that hunger, reduce feelings of fatigue, and make their struggle with weight loss more effective. Often associated with illness and disease due to higher fat content, they are excellent foods to include in a protein-type menu. So what about all the media that parallels high fat contents with illness? These foods contain saturated fat, which is not linked to the disorders you've probably associated it with. In fact, it's the fats found in refined carbohydrates, processed foods, and hydrogenated oils that have been directly linked to illness.

Important Points to Include in your Daily Meal Consumption:

Protein types need to eat a protein at every meal and with every snack. In fact, if they don't, they're likely to experience a spike in blood sugar and then a quick drop, which will leave someone with this metabolic type hungry and fatigued and with a craving for more carbohydrates.

Protein types need to eat small meals and more often, or plan healthy snacks in between meals. Snacks should also include a balance between proteins, fats, and carbohydrates in order to avoid the spikes and drops referenced above.

Protein types need to avoid an overabundance of carbohydrates like bread, pasta, and crackers. In fact, anything made from wheat can be very detrimental to protein types and their desired goals. Why? When it comes to losing weight, you want to avoid substances that break down into sugar, and this grain appears to break down faster than other grains, releasing large quantities of insulin. (Note: Insulin causes the body to store fat).

Protein types should also limit or avoid consuming too many fruits and fruit juices, even though in most instances they are considered healthy. Some fruits, like wheat, are converted to sugar within the bloodstream, which can lead to blood sugar fluctuations. That doesn't mean that you have to say "no" to all fruits and juices, just keep in mind those such as apple and avocadoes, which are high in fiber and low in sugar.

What if your metabolic type is that of Carbohydrate?

Carbohydrate Metabolic Types:

- Carbohydrate Types – Individuals within this category often forget about eating, which can actually be dangerous. Imagine this (true story): About sixteen years ago, before I knew anything about metabolic typing, I agreed to spend the weekend with a colleague of mine since her husband was going out of town. The first night was all right, as we'd gone out to dinner. However, by the second day around lunchtime, I was ravenous. Turns out, looking back, that she was definitely a "carb" type. In an effort to be a trouble-free guest, I was at the point of starvation before I finally mustered up the courage to inquire about food and eating. She stated when I asked, "Oh, I'm sorry – I don't eat much and in fact often forget to eat." Enough said.

  Individuals in this category typically forget to eat or choose not to eat, as they are often too busy to sit down and eat a square meal. Their metabolism, as a result, is directed into "starvation" mode, which leads to weight gain and obesity. Carb types often live on caffeine and desire teas, coffees, and foods that will provide them the rush that they need to get them through their day.

  Carbohydrate types love their sweets and will often crave cakes, cookies, pies, or starchy vegetables, which will sometimes show up later in life when these individuals are diagnosed as hypoglycemic, with diabetes, or perhaps find they are insulin resistant.

What do Carb types need in order to be successful in achieving their weight loss goals?

- Carb types need to eat a diet with more carbohydrates (70%) than proteins (20%) and should include healthy fats (10%) again, which should be derived from their protein source. Proteins for this metabolic type should include low-fat sources such as those one would find in poultry (white meat), or perch, bass, sole, cod, or haddock (the latter two are virtually fat-free). They can pull from a wide range of carbohydrates and eat much larger quantities than other metabolic groups.

  Individuals in this category are able to convert their carbohydrates into energy much more slowly than Protein types. However, this doesn't mean that they can consume countless numbers of them. Remember, carbohydrates stimulate the body's release of insulin, which is a fat-storing hormone, making weight loss virtually impossible for individuals within this category if they aren't careful.

Important Points to Consider if you are a Carbohydrate Metabolic type:

- Carbohydrate types must carefully select and make low-fat proteins a part of their daily dietary consumption. It's not imperative that you avoid proteins with a higher fat content altogether as that would be asking too much, but you should limit them, as they have been known to result in lethargy, depression and/or fatigue.
Dairy products are of special concern to individuals within this category, as often they aren't metabolized well. If you consume large amounts of this product, monitor your body's reaction to it and determine if you become lethargic or extremely fatigued afterwards.

  Low-starch vegetables are your best bet. Food items like salad greens, mustard or collard greens, spinach, celery, cauliflower, asparagus, and broccoli will fit nicely within your diet. Avoid carbs that are high-starch such as corn, carrots, potatoes, bread, pasta, and grains (wheat, rice, barley and oats).

  Legumes (beans, peas, and lentils) contain a specific protein that most individuals in this particular category cannot digest well, so monitor your body's response to them and eat accordingly.

  Last of all, monitor your consumption of nuts and seeds, as they contain too much fat for carbohydrate types. Although they provide an excellent source of protein for your snacks, you'll want to choose lean animal proteins for meals.

Mixed-Metabolic Types:

- Mixed Metabolic Types – It is essential if you fall into this group that you eat a balance of proteins (40%), carbohydrates (50%) and healthy fats (10%). Obviously, this is the easiest metabolic type to manage as you have more food choices. Keeping a healthy balance between protein and carbohydrate types, you'll find that your weight loss goals will be much easier to achieve.

  Individuals within this category are likely to be more like a roller coaster when it comes to eating habits. For instance, they might be ravenous at meals but not in between, and at other times they may have no appetite at all. Luckily, people within this category rarely have cravings for any particular food; however, if they eat too many carbohydrates and/or sugars, they may develop sugar cravings that normally wouldn't exist.

Like a Libra, balance is required, which means that high-fat and low-fat proteins must be incorporated into the diet, as well as both low and high-starch carbohydrates.

Individuals who are considered mixed type may favor one category (type) over the other. For instance, some persons may need more proteins than carbs within this category and therefore will need to more carefully monitor their weight loss.

Step Away from the Scale:

This may be hard to understand, but it isn't necessary to weigh yourself every single day. In fact, it can actually result in your attempts at weight loss being sabotaged. You probably know what I'm talking about, but just in case you don't, let me shine a light on it for you.

Suppose that you've been careful all week long, and then on Friday you weigh yourself and you've lost an astonishing 10 pounds. Yahoo!!! You think to yourself, "Let's celebrate." So you go out to dinner and a movie and you eat everything in sight. You've single-handedly sabotaged your weight loss plan, and instead of keeping the weight off, you've managed to throw your body's ability to metabolize your food effectively into a whirlwind. It practically has to start all over again to adjust to the curve ball you've just thrown its way.

Perhaps you've been extremely careful all week, making certain that you've eaten foods that you've been advised to eat according to the category that you fall within, and all of a sudden you've put on 10 pounds – WAIT!!!! Your body is perfectly capable of adding weight in the form of "water weight," depending upon your female cycle or other contributing factors. In fact, you may have added muscle mass to your body if you're exercising along with the dietary program. This sudden reflection in the scale may induce you to throw up your hands and quit. Don't do it. If you've been disciplined, you don't want to quit now. Evaluate – continue – and determine what may have altered your weight BEFORE quitting. Many times you'll be surprised.

If you, however, cannot avoid the scale no matter what, you'll want to ensure that you weigh yourself at the same time each day and that you're wearing the same clothes (or none at all). Depending upon the time of day, your body can reflect differences in body weight. So, if you cannot pass the scale by, you'll want to determine a specific time to weigh and then make certain that you do it following these tips, or you may get false results. I'd recommend that you weigh each morning (after emptying your bladder) before you get dressed to ensure that you're not adding the weight of clothes, shoes, etc., to the results.

Let's Talk About Fat:

Healthy Fats:

First of all, let me say, "All fat is not created equally." In fact, some fat is actually better for you than other types. Fat is known as a macronutrient and is necessary in a body's attempt to lose weight or fat that a body has accumulated. Dietary fat is an ally of a fit body, as it increases one's chance of getting fit and staying fit. In fact, the human body cannot survive without some fats, more specifically EFA's (Essential Fatty Acids). Alpha linolenic acid (ALA) is an omega-3 polyunsaturated fatty acid. Gamma linolenic acid (GLA) is an omega-6 unsaturated fatty acid.

These forms of fatty acids are closely related to the omega-3 fatty acids found in fish oils, which are called eicosapentaenoic acid or EPA and docosahexaenoic acid (DHA). So, what specifically does fat do for your body? It regulates our hormone levels; it is absolutely essential for healthy hair, skin, and nails; it helps to maintain a healthy heart and arteries; it maintains one's mood through prostaglandin modulation; controls our appetite by regulating our body's leptin response; it lowers a body's insulin response when we eat carbohydrates; and believe it or not, some FAT also burns fat! What? It's true! But you have to know which fat is good fat and which isn't. So let's review which fats our bodies need and which fats we should avoid:

- **Organic, unpasteurized butter & cream**: If you can get either of these from certified grass-fed cows, you'll benefit, as they contain fat-fighting enzymes and CLA, which is Conjugated Linoleic Acid and is believed to fight cancer.

- **Olives**: If you like olives, these little beauties are an excellent source of a healthy dose of monounsaturated fat, so load up your salad, or eat them right out of the jar. If, however, you aren't a real big fan, choose extra virgin olive oil, as it is a healthy alternative.

- **Peanuts and natural peanut butter**: Unless you are allergic, peanut butter is another excellent source of monounsaturated fat that should be included in your diet. Whether you prefer it right out of the jar, on a slice of bread, or on fruits or vegetables, it will provide your body with a healthy dose of fiber and plenty of healthy minerals.

- **Organic Flaxseed or Lignan Flaxseed Oil**: This is a purely vegetarian source of Omega-3 fatty acids, and an excellent antioxidant source in an oil form, but it cannot be used for cooking purposes. To get the most from this source, use it as an added ingredient to your salad dressing, or perhaps added to yogurt and/or cottage cheese. I've used ground flaxseed as a topping on my favorite ice cream or frozen yogurt, and have included it in my smoothies. Make sure to read the storage information as this product does expire.

- **Organic Virgin or Extra-Virgin Olive Oil**: Olive Oil has been promoted as one of the healthier oils on the market and is one that I include every day in my diet. You'll notice that I've recommended "organic" vs. the other oils on the market. Obviously, the more pure the product the more "whole" it actually is, and we know that whole foods are better for you. When talking about processing, the difference between extra-virgin olive oil and olive oil is the retention of the nutrients from the olive when it is pressed without an overabundance of salty brines, and it is even more concentrated. Of course, either form is loaded with hormone-regulating monounsaturated fat, but the extra-virgin contains higher antioxidant polyphenol levels that are antimicrobial and anti-inflammatory in nature, which suggests that they are or have been attributed to anti-cancer and being heart-friendly. An added perk is that they help to improve skin's clarity and glow by reducing oxidative stress, which is often attributed to excessive sun exposure and other factors.

- **Raw, unsalted Nuts, Nut Butters, and Cold-Pressed Nut Oils**: Excluding peanuts, the fats that are obtained from macadamias, pecans, pistachios, almonds, pecans, hazelnuts and walnuts are A-OK! In fact, they are excellent sources of protein and fiber with a healthy dose of monounsaturated fat, Vitamin E, and required minerals. If you aren't into eating a handful of nuts each day, try the butters, but you'll need to make certain that they aren't roasted before pressing. You'll always want to avoid commercial processing and can do this by simply pureeing them yourself. Any of the butters can be enjoyed with celery, apples, whole-grain crackers, or breads. Just remember your metabolic type.

- **Salmon (wild) or other fatty fish:** Probably one of my favorites, especially when cooked fresh (never frozen), Salmon is an excellent source of healthy fat while offering a high source of protein. When choosing Salmon, you want to purchase "wild" vs. farm raised in order to obtain the health benefitting Omega-3's, and powerful antioxidant and carotenoid, Astaxanthin. Although there are different options available to you, such as King, Sockeye, and Copper River, each beneficial in its own right, there are differences. For instance, the most significant difference is that Wild Salmon are "in the wild," meaning that they are able to eat a natural diet filled with algae and krill, which results in the "pink to red" tone of their bodies and being closer to 100% natural. Word of caution: Although Wild Salmon is definitely the best choice, due to the condition of our oceans, lakes, and rivers there is a higher level of PCB's (heavy metals), which are toxins. These toxins store themselves in fat, which means one should limit their intake of these fish to two days per week. If the natural form (fish) is not an option, you can also find a healthy supplement of purified fish or krill oil.

- **Organic, extra-Virgin Coconut Oil**: There it is again, "organic." Always choose this option when it is available, as it means less processed and containing more of the naturally derived and beneficial oil. While once upon a time we would have turned our back on this type of oil, as it has been associated with artery-clogging properties since it is a saturated fat, not all saturated fats are created equal. Obviously, keeping cholesterol levels under control is key, but some saturated fats, like coconut oil, are healthy oil and provide essential fatty acids, which actually provide energy and burn fat. The fatty acids found in coconut oil are delivered in the form of a medium chain triglyceride, or MCT, which is why it differs from the rest. These fatty acids behave as metabolic primers, turning up the heat in your internal fat-burning furnace, allowing it to burn fat quicker than other fats. Lauric Acid, which is a primary MCT found in coconut oil, includes some extremely potent antimicrobial properties. Like flaxseeds, check the storage instructions. Unrefined coconut oil is an excellent oil to cook with as it thrives under high heat conditions.

- **Fish Oil (Pharmaceutical Grade)**: Fish oils provide the same benefits as Wild Salmon and other fatty fish, but in a more concentrated formula of Omega-3 fatty acids. If you're one of the individuals that simply cannot tolerate the smell, texture, or taste of fish, this may be the route to take. Fish oils contain the long chain of Omega-3 fatty acids like DHA and EPA. They provide the body with the most anti-inflammatory and heart-healthy ingredients available in a supplement formula. Choose ONLY pharmaceutical grade so that you can insure that you receive the most pure formulation possible. Unfortunately, there are many *fish oils* available, but they aren't pure and can be dangerous, as they can contain PCB's and heavy metals that are obtained from the fish fat used for manufacturing the product.

- **Krill Oil (Neptune):** One supplement that you might want to consider, although not a food source, is Antarctic Pure Neptune Krill Oil. This extract, made from Antarctic Krill, is rich in cell membrane building blocks. It contains highly unsaturated phospholipids co-functionalized with Omega-3 fatty acids and has other desirable properties such as anti-aging benefits. It is known to provide protection enabling a healthy heart and joints and is promoted to reduce premenstrual symptoms. Neptune Krill Oil is cold-pressed from Antarctic Krill, which means, unlike fish oil, it is a concentrated formula of the purest Omega-3 fatty acids, DHA and EPA. Also, unlike other fish oils, it contains two powerful antioxidants, Astaxanthin and Canthaxanthin. Unlike Lycopene, Vitamin E, Coenzyme Q-10, Lutein, and Vitamin A, the free radical absorption capacity is equal to each of the above multiplied times four. In fact, it has thirty times more antioxidant power than Coenzyme Q-10 alone.

When choosing healthy fats to include within your daily diet, I'd recommend selecting and using at least 50% from the list above. Of course you'll want to include other fats, such as those that are found within other protein sources like your meat, poultry, and dairy fat, but you'll know to limit those fats in lieu of more healthy "healing" fats.

Now that we've reviewed the "healthy" fats that we should choose from on a daily dietary basis, we need to become familiar with "unhealthy" fats and fats that we should avoid as often as possible. Unfortunately, there are many fats that are simply unhealthy to the human body. In order to understand what these fats are, you need to understand how they are manufactured or processed.

Saturated Fat:

What are saturated fats and what do you really know about them? More than likely you've been told that saturated fats are "bad" and that you should avoid them if at all possible. You've probably also been told that they are contributors to high cholesterol and heart disease. Well, you might be surprised to learn that before "hydrogenated fats and oils" we had saturated fats and oils derived from dairy and meat products in our daily diets almost exclusively. We used butter for baking, frying, and other needs such as a topping on our toast, plopped on our potatoes (whatever type they were) and to season our foods (along with fatback).

Did you also know that heart disease was extremely rare before the 1920's? In fact, until around the 1950's, people simply didn't suffer from clogged arteries or heart disease like they did after that time. By 1955, heart disease became the leading cause of death among Americans and today, at least 40% of all deaths can be attributed to heart disease.

The question that I must ask is, if saturated fat consumption actually decreased between 1910 and 1970 from 83% to 62%, how then did the health risks associated with saturated fats increase? In fact, during the last eighty years, the consumption of dietary cholesterol has increased by only 1%. During the same period of time, the average intake of dietary vegetable oils (either margarine, shortening like Crisco, and refined oils) increased by a whopping 400% and the consumption of refined sugar and processed foods increased by 60%.

Based on the numbers provided above, I'm inclined to believe that saturated fats have been falsely accused. What about you? Ask a manufacturer and they will certainly beg to differ, but the numbers speak volumes.

Do you remember earlier when we were discussing "healthy" oils? Well, coconut oil is one of them, but it is also known to be a saturated fat. Guess what? It contains NO trans-fat and is rich in lauric acid, which again is a wonderful natural provider of antiviral, antibacterial, and antifungal properties. In fact, Dr. Al Sears, M.D., states, "The saturated fat found in coconut oil is a unique fat that helps prevent heart disease, helps to build up the immune system, and does not turn into fat in your body."

In fact, your body actually recognizes it and knows how to metabolize it instead of storing it in your fat cells, plus it speeds up your metabolism, which means burning fat faster – and who doesn't want that? Another doctor, Joseph Mercola, D.O., states that, "Coconut oil is truly the healthiest oil you can consume," and encourages people to find and use virgin coconut oil for all of their cooking needs in order to experience the difference for themselves.

Unhealthy Fats:

Unhealthy fats come in many processed foods and under many different "scientific" names. For instance, next time you're in the grocery store, pick up a package of cookies, chips, margarine, or other pre-packaged snack and food items and read the label. You'll notice trans fats or perhaps trans-fatty acids (TFAs). These are referred to as hydrogenated oils or partially hydrogenated oils. These are the types of fats that should be avoided.

When reading labels, which I truly hope that you do or begin to do, if you see the phrase or words "hydrogenated," put it back, take a deep breath, and walk away from the shelf. It is the process of hydrogenation that you should understand, and then it will make sense to you. When you take unsaturated oil and "zap it" with high-pressure hydrogen, you turn the oil into saturated fat. The best example that I can provide that you might be able to envision is taking vegetable oil, zapping it, and tada - you have margarine.

It is when you take a product and make it more shelf-stable with a higher melting point. In order to do this, the oil is washed, bleached, and deodorized and then brought to a boil with a metal catalyst such as nickel, zinc, or copper. The hydrogen gas is "zapped" through the liquid mixture and you end up with the final product. Partially hydrogenated products would be something similar to margarine, thickened salad dressings, or products that don't separate within the bottle.

Hydrogenated would be more along the lines of Crisco shortening. What occurs during the process is that you've turned what was a natural fat into an unnatural trans-fat, which the body does not recognize and therefore treats it as a toxin, storing it within fat cells and your arteries. In fact, the molecular structure of a trans-fat is more similar to that of plastic than to a normal, natural fatty acid. So why do so many foods contain them?

Hydrogenated fats are better alternatives for manufacturers in that they provide two major economic advantages over natural saturated fats.

1) They are cheaper to manufacture than products containing saturated fats.
2) They have a longer shelf life, meaning that they can occupy space on the supermarket shelves longer than products that expire.

They are also used more frequently in fast food and restaurant establishments because they can tolerate higher heat, often used when frying foods and again, because they last longer.

Don't be fooled when you are reading labels, either, because manufacturers have a way of making hydrogenated oils appear less unhealthy than they are. For instance, when you read the label, it may say, "cholesterol-free," which makes you let down your guard. But wait!!! Looking a little closer you'll see plenty of artery-clogging saturated fat.

Hydrogenated fats also harbor another kind of fat that exists outside the saturated and unsaturated categories… these are trans-fatty acids or trans-fats. They derived these special names because the hydrogenation process transports hydrogen atoms across the fat molecules, delivering them to a new location. Trans-fats, as described by Dr. Udo Erasmus, are "molecules that have their head on backwards." In fact, he describes trans-fats as being as bad for or worse for your arteries than saturated fats.

Many studies have been conducted over the years on trans-fats and they've consistently reflected increases in cholesterol levels in the blood of the participants studied. Unfortunately for all of us, in 1999 the United States modified label laws, dropping the stipulation that food manufacturers must include information about trans-fats in nutrition labeling. In other words, "Buyer Beware!"

There's more about trans-fats that we need to discover before we can move on. We're all familiar with the term "Saturated Fats," and for many of us this term may make you take a deep breath or sigh a little heavier than normal. The truth is there's more to this type of fat than meets the eye and we need to learn more about it.

Trans-fats are included in almost every pre-packaged food purchased and offer very little in the form of nutrition to the unsuspecting consumer. The only thing that we can honestly say is that trans-fats will provide one with a source of energy. We can also say, as consumers have learned and can attest to over the years, foods containing trans-fats are often more expensive – potato chips, cookies, and other snack foods or prepared meals. Why? Manufacturers can produce foods cheaper, which will last longer, and at a price consumers will wince at but pay if it makes life more convenient. But is it really convenient?

Butter, delicious, all-natural butter that our grandparents (and even some of our parents) made themselves on the farm got a bad reputation as a saturated fat full of cholesterol. So what did manufacturers do? They developed margarine. Do you want the good news or bad news first? Let's start with some details. When manufacturers chemically modify food, lots of unanticipated problems often result. This, of course, is especially true of hydrogenated fatty acids as described earlier.

- Hydrogenated fats, once consumed, behave biochemically in the body just like saturated fats… Hmm… so, what they're saying is that margarine acts the same within the body as butter??? Go figure!

- Trans-fats are known to elevate blood cholesterol levels similarly to saturated fats.

- Trans-fats raise LDL (bad) cholesterol levels.

- Trans-fats reduce HDL (good) cholesterol levels and raise the bad cholesterol levels in the process, which equals double-trouble.

- Trans-fats have been linked to decreased production of natural anti-inflammatory prostaglandins.

- Eating nutritionally worthless hydrogenated fats may decrease a person's consumption of other fats and essential fatty acids that are important for growth and optimum function of vital organs such as the brain. If you have young children, this is especially alarming if they are frequent visitors of fast food restaurants specializing in processed and deep fat-fried foods and snacks.

- Trans-fats or hydrogenated fats may interfere with a body's ability to metabolize fats that are good for it. These fats may damage cell membranes on vital structures such as the brain and nerve cells. Cell membranes contain many receptor sites for fat molecules, so when the "healthy" fatty acid arrives it is processed in order to contribute to the membrane. However, biochemical imposters may squeeze into a space that doesn't know how to process it, therefore the body cannot get what it needs. It is moved through the body trying to find the proper location, and unfortunately may damage or cause harm to other locations. It may also weaken the body's ability to accept and process what cell membranes need and block out what the body needs. Through this process, the body may be susceptible to chronic degenerative diseases. In the medical community, "fake fats" are now becoming labeled "the silent killer."

- Trans-fatty acids have been associated with other health problems, including decreased testosterone, abnormal sperm production, and prostate disease in men; obesity, immune system depression, and even diabetes.

Here are a few helpful charts, which may make it easier to choose good fats rather than bad fats. Fats in the charts below contain a minimum of 80% unsaturated fats. Most contain some essential fatty acids, and all contribute to the health and well-being of the mind and body.

FOOD	COMMENT
Human milk	Richest overall source of healthy fats.
Algae oil	Richest source of DHA.
Flax seeds, flax oil	Richest source of essential fatty acids and DHA.
Fish (cold-water, especially Atlantic salmon and tuna)	Coldwater fish, especially salmon and tuna are, like flax, rich sources of DHA.
Seeds (sunflower, pumpkin)	Rich source of essential omega 6 fatty acids, mostly unsaturated fats.
Canola oil	Ranks second to flax oil as the oil richest in essential fatty acids, especially DHA.
Soy products (e.g., soy milk, tofu, tempeh)	Rich in essential omega 3 and omega 6 fatty acids, similar to fish oils. Also, contains lecithin; can reduce cholesterol.
Olive oil	Mostly unsaturated fats.
Nuts	Almonds and walnuts contain 90 percent unsaturated fats; cashews are low in total fat and it is mostly unsaturated.
Monounsaturated Fats	
Peanut butter	Mostly unsaturated fats; buy organic and unhydrogenated. Also, good source of protein. Healthy alternatives to peanut butter are soybean butter, sesame seed butter, and cashew butter.
Hummus (a spread made from chickpeas)	Approximately 85 percent unsaturated fats, plus good source of protein, folic acid, many vitamins and minerals, and no cholesterol.
Wheat germ	Mostly unsaturated fat, plus a rich source of vitamins, minerals and proteins.

Fats in this category contain a balance of saturated and unsaturated fatty acids, which, if eaten in moderation, contribute to the health and well-being of the body. Look for low-fat varieties. These goods are rich sources of other nutrients as well.

FOODS	COMMENT
Yogurt (low fat)	Like all dairy products, mostly saturated fats.
Milk (1 or 2 percent)	Around 50 percent of the fat content of whole milk.
Egg	More unsaturated than saturated fats; yolk is high in cholesterol; use only egg white if you are cholesterol sensitive.
Beef (sirloin, trimmed)	High cholesterol, around 50-50 saturated and unsaturated fats.
Turkey (breast, skinless)	Around 50-50 saturated and unsaturated fats.
Veal (loin)	About 50-50 saturated and unsaturated fats
Cocoa butter	Even though it is a saturated fat, it is metabolized like a monounsaturated fat similar to those contained in olive oil.

If you could eliminate all of the fats in this category you would be healthier for it. Any nutrient that might be in any of these fats could be obtained from other fats with better nutritional credentials.

FOODS	COMMENT
Tallow (chicken or beef)	Ninety percent saturated fats
Lard	High in saturated fatty acids
Palm-kernel oil	Mostly saturated fats. Contains palmitoleic acid, a fat, which, if eaten in excess, can interfere with essential fatty acid metabolism.
Coconut oil	Over 90 percent saturated fats
"Hydrogenated," or "partially hydrogenated"	Tops the list of fats that are bad for you.
Margarines	High in hydrogenated fats, especially those with a lot of coconut, palm-kernel, and hydrogenated oils.
Shortening	Especially those with lard, hydrogenated oils, palm kernel, coconut oils, or tallow.
Cottonseed oil	More unsaturated than saturated fat, but usually hydrogenated and may contain pesticide residues.

Last, but certainly not least on your journey and education about fats is about the type of fat most of us cringe when we hear – saturated fats. However, after reading what you've just read about hydrogenated or trans-fats, I'm sure you'll agree they aren't as frightening after all.

Let's Get Cooking with Fat(s):

I know you're shaking your head and wondering if you heard me correctly. Yes, you did! I'm going to share with you some very important information about cooking with fats that everyone needs to know. Whether you're rarely in the kitchen or are responsible for preparing meals for your family, friends, or loved ones on a regular basis, it is important to understand that different types of fat react to temperature in many different ways. In other words, different fats have a different volatility (smoke) point when heated, and knowing which fats will respond best for the purposes that you're using them will guarantee success in the kitchen.

Let me explain. Every fat will begin to smoke, become discolored, and decompose, damaging any and all fatty acid content that is contained in the source product. When you overheat fat to this point, it becomes spoiled and unhealthy.

There are two fat sources that are recommended for cooking:

1) Virgin (unrefined) coconut oil: When shopping for coconut oil, it is best to find oil that is in its purest form. Coconut oil, although saturated, is excellent for cooking at extremely high heat. Plus, because it is a medium-chain fatty acid (MCFA), it goes immediately to the liver, where it is converted to energy instead of being stored as fat.

2) Raw/Organic Butter: You may have to look a little harder to find it in the supermarket or make your own (my preference), but this is the perfect fat for cooking at medium-high heat. It, like coconut oil, stays chemically stable up to 375 degrees, which means that you'll end up with a healthier, more delicious end product. It is also one of the healthiest whole foods that you can include in your diet, even though it contains high levels of saturated fat.

Other fats that can be used for cooking are of course, olive oil. It is low in saturated fat and high in monounsaturated fat. This product is best consumed raw, such as sprinkled over a salad or vegetable, OR for light sautéing over medium heat. When purchasing olive oil, it is best if you choose partly cloudy oil with a yellow tint, as that indicates it is unrefined, which means that the healthy elements have NOT been filtered out.

Fats that you'll want to avoid in the kitchen, but unfortunately so many of us have been led to believe they are healthier for us and the way to go (and more than likely are in your pantry now) are:

- Trans-fats (hydrogenated oils) like safflower, sunflower, shortening (Crisco), vegetable, corn, and soybean oils.

To make things a little easier for you, I'm attaching a chart, which includes both refined and unrefined oils (fats) used for cooking. It will provide their volatility (or smoke points) so that you'll know what temperatures are best for each.

Cooking With Oils

Low heat = 275° to 325° F • **Medium heat** = 325° to 350° F • **Medium-high heat** = 350° to 400° F • **Very high heat** = 400° to 495° F — Please note, oil availability may vary by store.

Oil	Raw	Low heat	Med. heat	Med. High heat	Very high heat	Characteristics and uses
Almond, refined	X	X	X	X	X	Pure, clean flavor and a high-heat wonder. Smoke point 495° F.
Avocado (expeller-pressed), refined	X	X	X	X	X	Lovely texture, wonderful for searing meat, whipped potatoes and stir-fries. Smoke point 450° F.
Avocado (cold-pressed), unrefined	X	X	X	X	X	Lovely texture, wonderful for searing meat, whipped potatoes and stir-fries. Smoke point 500° F.
Canola (medium-high heat), refined	X	X	X	X		Neutral flavor, all-purpose, good for baking. Smoke point 425° F. May be genetically modified if not organic.
Canola, unrefined	X	X				Mild flavor, may be genetically modified if not organic.
Coconut (virgin/extra virgin), unrefined		X	X			Lovely for cakes, pie crusts, light sautéing. Cholesterol-free. Smoke point 280° to 350° F.
Ghee		X	X	X		Wonderful in sauces, with lobster or crab, and for quick frying.
Grape seed (expeller-pressed), refined	X	X	X	X	X	Clean, neutral taste. Smoke point 485° F.
Hazelnut, unrefined	X					Rich flavor. Drizzle on food or use for dipping bread. Potential allergen.
Macadamia nut (cold-pressed), unrefined	X					Nutty, buttery flavor and higher in Monounsaturates than olive oil.
Olive (extra virgin), unrefined	X	X				Ideal for salads, raw foods, pesto and dipping bread. Smoke point 325° F.
Olive (extra light/original), refined	X	X	X	X		Mild and tolerant of low heat. Smoke point 460° F.

Oil	Raw	Low heat	Med. heat	Med. High heat	Very high heat	Characteristics and uses
Peanut (expeller-pressed, vitamin E added), refined	X	X	X	X		Adds flavor to lightly cooked foods and cold dishes. Smoke point 212° to 400° F. Potential allergen.
Peanut (high oleic), refined	X	X	X	X	X	Neutral flavor for tempura, fish and stir-fries. Smoke point 450° F. Potential allergen.
Safflower (high heat), refined	X	X	X	X	X	Mild flavor for high-heat cooking. Smoke point 450° F.
Safflower, unrefined	X					Delicate flavor.
Sesame, refined	X	X	X	X	X	Adds smoky flavor to seared meats, stir-fries. Smoke point 445° F.
Sesame, unrefined (including toasted)	X					Aromatic, nutty, best in dressings and sauces.
Sunflower (high oleic), refined	X	X	X	X	X	Nearly neutral flavor. Smoke point 450° F.
Sunflower (expeller-pressed), refined	X	X	X	X	X	Multi-purpose. Smoke point 460° F.
Sunflower (cold-pressed), unrefined	X					Rich flavor, best in cold dishes.
Vegetable shortening (palm fruit), refined		X	X	X		Good for cakes, pie crusts, sautés. Not hydrogenated.
Walnut, refined	X	X	X	X		Adds character to salads, marinades and sautés. Smoke point 400° F. Potential allergen.

Low heat = 275° to 325° F • **Medium heat** = 325° to 350° F • **Medium-high heat** = 350° to 400° F • **Very high heat** = 400° to 495° F — Please note, oil availability may vary by store.

I hope that this clears up any misconceptions about your "fat" choices in the kitchen and provides you a tool for choosing the proper oils for whatever your cooking needs (remember, natural, unrefined, raw are always best).

CHAPTER SIX
ORGANIC FOODS (WHOLE) VS. THE OTHER OPTIONS

Not everybody believes, "The body is your temple. Keep it pure and clean for the soul to reside in." ~B.K.S. Iyengar, *Yoga: The Path to Holistic Health.* I sure do, because as it is so eloquently expressed by Jim Rohn, "Take care of your body. It's the only place you have to live." That pretty much says it all in my opinion. And, what you put into your body and the manner in which you treat it will definitely determine whether your temple is built of bricks or straw in the long run.

Organic foods (and products) will provide you the best choices for feeding and nourishing your temple. Why? Organic food products are grown and/or raised without using synthetic pesticides, herbicides, fungicides, or fertilizers. What is synthetic? Simply put – chemically formulated. Think about it, if you have the option of ingesting organic products that don't have chemical residues on the outside, which ultimately leech into the fruit or vegetable, then you won't be eating pesticides, herbicides, fungicides, or fertilizers. Why would you want to?

Unfortunately, consumers in the United States are exposed to so many chemically formulated products via their food sources that it is alarmingly scary. Over 2 billion pounds of pesticides (poison) are sprayed on crops to offset poor farming practices – easy way mentality. Put another way, "Why do sit-ups when you can purchase Contour Abs to do the work for you while you sit and watch television?" These chemicals, once ingested, can alter our body's behavior and manner of processing the foods consumed in many ways.

So, let's talk about why organic food choices are better for you and why you should choose organic vs. conventionally farmed foods.

Why Choose Organic?

Well, first and foremost, choosing organic means that you're choosing NOT to purchase products that have been chemically treated with pesticides and other toxins that can ultimately affect your health and well-being. To me, it just makes sense. To others, not so much! Let me explain this concept in a way that just might alter your thoughts about organic foods vs. the other options.

In organic farming, everything is done naturally. The soil is treated and/or composted from organic materials so that you get the best quality soil in which to grow your foods. Helpful insects are used to manage other pests, which are not. However, with conventionally farmed fruits and vegetables, pesticides, which belong to the halogenated hydrocarbon family of toxins such as DDE, PCB, dieldrin, and chlordane, are used to treat certain funguses and rid the plants of pests, which ultimately destroy or minimize the crops. Chemicals such as these will last a lifetime in the environment, meaning that they'll still exist when I'm long gone and my children's children are grown. A perfect example would be the chemical DDT, which was banned thirty years ago, but which can still be found in root vegetables like potatoes and carrot crops harvested today.

These chemicals, when ingested, cannot be processed properly by the liver. Our bodies have a difficult time detoxifying and eliminating these compounds, which ultimately are stored in our fat cells. Once inside the body, these toxins take on a similar role to that of the hormone estrogen, which is now suspected to be a contributing factor in the ever-increasing epidemic of estrogen-related health problems such as breast cancer. If that isn't enough, these chemical toxins have also been linked to the development of lymphomas, pancreatic cancer, and leukemia, and play a significant role in the low sperm count and reduced fertility in men.

Finally, it might surprise you to learn that those who are at the greatest risk of developing complications associated with pesticide toxins are our innocent children. They consume more food in relation to their body weight and eat more of the highly toxic foods such as fresh fruit, fruit juices, and vegetables than do adults. In fact, the Consumers Union advises parents to avoid purchasing and serving conventionally farmed products that contain higher levels of residue such as cantaloupes, fresh, canned, or frozen green beans, winter squash, strawberries, Mexican-grown tomatoes, and pears, while the University of Washington added apples to the list.

How do you know if the Produce is Organic?

When shopping for safe, organic products, you may feel that you are at the mercy of the merchant. That is simply not the case, as there is an organization in place in order to protect the consumer and ensure that we are getting the products for which we are paying.

The National Organic Program was established to ensure that the production, processing, and certification of foods labeled organic meet the comprehensive standards in place. Large farming or processing operations must be certified, while smaller farms' uncertified organic must follow certain labeling standards and procedures. For individuals who are unfamiliar with the different levels of organic products, I'm going to provide a list below to assist you when you are shopping.

- "100% organic" – No synthetic ingredients are allowed by law.
- "Organic" – At least 95% of the ingredients are organically produced.
- "Made with Organic Ingredients" – At least 70% of the ingredients are organic; the other 30% are from a list approved by the USDA.
- "Free-range" or "free-roaming" – Animals had an undetermined amount of daily outdoor access. This label does not provide much information about the product.
- "Natural" or "All Natural" – Doesn't mean organic. No standard definition, except for meat or poultry products, which may not contain any artificial flavoring, colors, chemical preservatives or synthetic ingredients. Claims aren't checked.

When it comes to meat, including poultry and eggs, you are what you eat. In other words, if you're consuming animal products, depending upon what they were fed, you'll benefit to the level or degree of the foods they ate. With cattle raised on the range, they'll eat wild grasses, whereas commercially raised cattle are more often fed low-quality or inexpensive grains in an effort to fatten them up, and sometimes there will be an added growth hormone in their foods as well. Now, what you may not realize is that cattle were NOT intended to eat grain, they were intended to eat grass. Therefore, they frequently become ill, requiring the administration of antibiotics that will then be consumed when you eat meats.

Likewise, poultry and swine are typically raised commercially in small pens referred to as "factory" farms, and often in their own feces. These animals do not often see the light of day. They are administered absurd doses of antibiotics and growth hormones to increase the rate of growth and to keep them alive. This detail alone should encourage or inspire consumers to seek free-range organic chicken and pork and spend the extra dollars in order to do so.

Finally, an egg is only as healthy as the quality of life the chicken that laid it lived. Therefore, if you want good eggs, you'll want to find cartons labeled organic, free-range, antibiotic, and hormone-free. Keeping this in mind, the healthier the egg, the higher the levels of Omega-3 fatty acids that will result. In fact, eggs are known to be the most well-balanced natural food for human consumption. However, in order to enjoy the health benefits, the eggs must be organic. Why? Commercially raised chickens/eggs are high in Omega-6 fats, which cause inflammation within the body and increase the risk of heart disease.

Cost Prohibitive – Which Costs More? Your Health or Your Groceries?

Obviously, organic foods more often than not reflect a higher cost. This is because the farming procedures and practices are much more labor intensive. Farmers actually go the extra yard to ensure that their produce and/or farm animals are toxin-free for consumers to enjoy. What does this mean? Well, for one thing, organic farmers do not produce as much quantity as commercial farmers. Secondly, they will hand weed their crops in lieu of pesticides and herbicides, which the commercial farms will often overuse to make their jobs easier. Finally, because they do not receive government subsidies, they must rely on their products to generate an income enough to support themselves, their employees, and their farms.

Short term, one could consider the organic foods to be more expensive than conventionally farmed products. However, in the long run, which is less expensive – a healthy individual or one who requires medical attention due to toxins consumed over the years? Medical care is not cheap these days and increases each and every day – especially if you don't have suitable medical coverage. So I suppose the question that you must ask yourself is, "Is my health worth the extra dollars spent now vs. the medical bills that I'll be required to pay when my income is solely dependent upon my retirement and Social Security benefits?" Well? Or, you can plant your own fruits and vegetables and harvest them yourself to insure what chemicals, if any, aren't applied, keeping them toxin free. You can purchase seeds, plant them, and then harvest the vegetables for much less than you can purchase these foods in the store or farmers market. I've been planting my own organic garden since my children were infants to ensure that what they consumed was healthy, toxin free, and completely within my control, and I was able to do so in a space no larger than 4 feet by 8 feet. I built a raised bed, allowing full control of the space and making it impossible for wild animals to eat the foods I'd grown for my family.

Put another way, if you were diagnosed with an illness that required special medical equipment, attention, and medications in order for you to enjoy your life, would you say, "It's too expensive," and opt out of the necessary items, or would you make certain that the items were available to you so that you could enjoy your life? Organic foods are the items necessary to ensure that you will enjoy a long and healthy life. Isn't it worth it?

The good news is, if you are living on a budget, which most of America is these days, you can still eat organic foods. You simply have to evaluate and/or consider which foods are more tainted with toxins than others. For instance, if you know that commercially farmed green beans are more toxic than onions, choose and purchase the healthier commercially farmed products (onions) and spend your money on organic green beans. This way, you're able to benefit both ways.

Having shared this information, let me now address food items that should ALWAYS be purchased organic if they are available in your area. This information is based on analysis compiled by The EWG Working Group. Please note items referenced in **BOLD** letters are indicative of foods that are more laden with pesticides.

- Apples
- Bell Peppers
- **CELERY**
- Cherries
- Grapes (especially if they are imported)
- Lettuce
- **PEACHES**
- Pears
- Potatoes
- **RASPBERRIES (red)**
- **SPINACH**
- Strawberries

The items referenced below are not often associated with multiple pesticides, which mean that they can be purchased from commercial farms.

- **Avocado**
- **Banana**
- **Broccoli**

- **Cauliflower**
- **Corn**
- **Eggplant**
- **Kiwi**
- **Mango**
- **Papaya**
- Pineapple
- Sweet Peas

So, when choosing between what foods to purchase organically and which are safe to purchase from commercially produced items, go organic on the first list and conventional on the second.

CHAPTER SEVEN
THE ABC's ON THE FOODS WE EAT

A trip to the supermarket can really be an eye-opening experience. If you're a label reader, you know what I'm talking about. If you're not, you may want to hop on board and become one along with me. Most consumers will place products into their carts based on a few factors: 1) what their parents purchased when they were growing up; 2) what advertisers have promoted as being the "newest," "greatest," and "healthiest" product on the market; 3) what the kids want and desire; 4) the easiest items to prepare. When selecting items, there are quite a few more important factors to consider. In fact, they just might save your life by helping you to eliminate the possibility of a lifetime of illness and disease.

Let's address many items that are available that we might want to consider a little more carefully the next time we shop:

Alcohol:

I know I probably sound like your wife, husband, or parent, but there are truly many factors alcohol affects that you should know if you're trying to lose weight. In fact, this is one topic that I actually do not enjoy commenting on, since so many individual enjoy their drinks. Unfortunately, however, I cannot share the details about healthy weight-loss without mentioning them to you. Obviously, you can make the decision whether or not the information is relevant to you and your weight-loss goals.

Many of us believe that certain types of alcohol are beneficial to our overall health – especially when it comes to the heart. We've been told that it can reduce cholesterol, calm the nerves, reduce stress, etc. The truth is, however, that alcohol is a high-calorie beverage that is actually toxic to the liver and therefore does nothing to assist in one's weight-loss efforts.

Mixed drinks, one of the more popular drink choices, are actually loaded with calories – anywhere from 100 – 250 calories, in fact. But what's worse is that when people are consuming alcoholic beverages they don't give much consideration to the amount of food that they're consuming. In fact, certain alcoholic beverages actually make individuals crave certain foods, and those foods are actually choices that we should avoid, like those containing excess carbohydrates and sugar.

The human body treats alcohol like a toxin when it comes to processing the calories consumed. Although it is considered a carbohydrate, the body doesn't process it like other carbohydrates that people enjoy. Alcohol contains 7 calories per gram, whereas other carbohydrates contain 4 calories per gram. When alcohol is introduced to your system, the liver attempts to process the calories associated with it before all others. Consequently, while the body is waiting to process the other calories consumed, the body naturally stores them away in the fat cells, which is not a good thing if you're attempting to lose weight. Besides, who wants to consume a beverage made of fermented wheat, barley, grapes, and other carbohydrates like potatoes?

Dairy Products:

We all have heard the saying "Got Milk" and know how it motivates us to run to the refrigerator and pour a tall glass, but do you know what you're actually consuming when you're drinking pasteurized milk? Once upon a time, milk was considered a primary staple in our daily diet – today, not so much. In fact, the modification of the daily recommended requirements from three servings to none speaks volumes. Today's milk isn't what it used to be. In fact, it is nowhere near the wholesome drink or snack that most of us grew up drinking. Let's review why.

Remember in the previous section when we discussed commercially farmed products and the toxins that are associated with produce and meats that are generated from them? Well, dairy is one of those products that have been tainted so much that it's more harmful than good. In fact, it makes me question the slogan, "Milk – it does the body Good," because it actually does not.

A Little History:

First, a little history lesson. As a college student I was heavily involved with IFAS (Institute of Food and Agricultural Science), which was part of the university's College of Agriculture. I actually lived at the Dairy Research unit, which was used as a teaching tool for students (and the government) to discover which farming practices would produce more milk, less infection, etc. Well, I was shocked at the practices that were used to increase overall milk production and the practices used during the milking process. But that's not where it stopped.

After graduation, I married and moved to a commercial dairy farm with my husband. He was the assistant manager at one of two locations, and therefore I got first-hand knowledge of the practices and procedures used in the industry. From an overabundance of growth hormones, antibiotics, and pesticides, to poor nutrition supplied to the animals, I learned more in that year than many will learn in a lifetime. Needless to say, I won't drink commercially produced milk.

Raw Milk vs. Pasteurized Milk:

Before pasteurization in the early 1900's, milk was served unpasteurized and non-homogenized from free-range grass-fed cattle. It was served in its most natural form. Although it can be difficult to obtain these days, many co-ops still make it possible for families to get their hands on it through partial ownership of a cow from which the milk is obtained. (It's illegal to sell unprocessed/raw milk in many states, but if you own the cow – you can drink all the milk you want). Raw dairy is expensive to produce due to the sensitive farming practices, and most consumers aren't willing to pay the price when they can purchase pasteurized milk and dairy products for less. The health advantages are worth the extra money spent. Let me now share with you why.

Pasteurization was originally designed to treat milk in the event it was tainted with tuberculosis, botulism, and other diseases so it wouldn't be transferred to humans through its consumption. These days, it isn't necessary to kill these types of diseases or bacteria, but milk is still pasteurized, which actually has proven to be ineffective at killing the very things it was pasteurized to destroy in the first place. In fact, pasteurization doesn't occur at a temperature high enough to kill bacteria that cause typhoid and tuberculosis. As a matter of fact, there have been incredibly high rates of Salmonella contaminated milk after pasteurization.

Unpasteurized milk has not been linked to illnesses, especially at the same level or degree of processed milk. Why? A bacterium within raw milk actually protects it from pathogens that can lead to illness and disease in humans. Pasteurization kills the beneficial bacteria that is naturally produced and therefore makes it impossible for the "natural" process of disease control to take place. Instead, we're left with a product that when it has "expired" or it has gone bad can actually be dangerous to consume, whereas raw milk will turn to buttermilk or sour cream.

Conventional / Commercially Farmed Milk:

Today, milk is processed in so many different ways to insure that it is "safe" – a questionable term - to market commercially. From transportation from the dairy farm to pasteurization, milk's natural form is altered so much that it truly isn't the healthy beverage that we enjoyed long ago. Pasteurization destroys milk's natural germicidal elements as well as most of the healthy enzymes that are necessary for the proper digestion. In fact, as a result of this processing, many people have become lactose intolerant. In order to still enjoy the taste of dairy (although it's the modified taste they're attempting to enjoy) they are then motivated to use non-dairy products, which end up causing problems far worse than the dairy products they're attempting to replace.

To make matters worse, during the pasteurization process, 50% of milk's calcium becomes unstable. The human body cannot assimilate it, and therefore the "healthy" benefits become moot. Not only is the lack of calcium a major contributor to osteoporosis in the United States, but the synthetic vitamin D2 is toxic and linked to heart disease, and vitamin D3 is difficult for the body to absorb.

Homogenization:

Yet another practice of conventionally processed milk, homogenization is intended to reduce the size of fat molecules contained in raw milk. Why is this significant? When the fat molecules are processed to reduce their size, they are then able to bypass the digestion process, which increases the changes of incomplete protein digestion that takes place in the small intestine. It allows some of the milk proteins to be absorbed into the bloodstream, which can result in a sensitization of the immune system, causing an allergy and intolerance to milk.

Growth Hormones and Antibiotics:

Now I will visit a topic that everyone should be concerned with when it comes to choosing healthy products for themselves and their families. I touched upon it briefly in the little history lesson, but feel as if you need to know the facts.

Large (and small) dairy operations supply the larger companies with their product – raw milk. Unfortunately, it is the practices that these commercially run dairy farms implement that "taint" our milk and other dairy products that we purchase.

Dairy farms earn their money when they sell their milk to the large processing plants (and when they sell calves to meat distributors.) So it stands to reason that the more milk that's produced, the higher the profits the smaller farms earn. In order to increase the milk supply that the farm has to sell, they must alter the natural milk production of the cow. In most instances, a dairy cow will produce milk for about 12 weeks after calving. Although it is a strain on the cow's organs to produce milk as quickly as the farmer would like, many farmers are only concerned with the output of milk. This is done through the administration of growth hormones (rBGH – recombinant bovine growth hormone). This enables the farmer to increase milk production from 8 – 12 weeks.

Through the process of extending and increasing the cow's natural ability to produce milk, the cow becomes 80% more susceptible to infections. One such infection is mastitis, which is infection of the udder. Now, for those of you who don't know what an udder is, it is the part of the cow that contains the milk before it is processed through a "teat" by an automatic or robotic milking machine. When an udder/teat becomes infected, farmers are forced to administer antibiotics so that the cow's milk can still be used. If this happens, the antibiotic is introduced to the milk supply, which is then processed for humans to drink.

One last practice that I found alarming was the number of farms that were too cheap to use proper procedures and products (germicides) for cleansing the cow's teat before milking. Cows are penned and have a tendency to lie down in pastures, where they are exposed to many elements, even feces. Before a cow is milked, for sanitary purposes the cow must have the teats cleaned. This can be done many different ways, but unfortunately the most common method is not always the safest – for the consumer. It is common practice for farms to use bleach, in which they will dip the cow's teat before attaching the robotic milking machine.

For anyone that knows about bleach, it is a registered pesticide with the Environmental Protection Agency. Yes, many people use it in their homes for cleaning purposes – and I suppose that is their right. But, to use a toxic chemical on an animal (who doesn't have a choice) to sanitize and/or clean a teat BEFORE it is then attached to a machine to extract the milk (and toxic bleach residue) that consumers will then consume should be illegal. Unfortunately, farms get away with this practice and the consumer suffers the consequences.

Health Risks:

You may be wondering how the U.S. FDA would allow such practices to be implemented when consumers ultimately become the "guinea pig." The U. S. Food and Drug Administration suggest that there is no difference between milk from cows treated with growth hormones and untreated cows (Chek 2004, 67). Unfortunately, because it's big money business, many things aren't made public. One company did, in fact, conduct a study, and found that ALL of the cows that received rBGH got cancer whether they received the hormone intravenously or ingested it orally. (Chek 2004, 67).

Grains:

From cavemen to modern man, our diets have changed dramatically. Gone are the days when we were forced to capture or slay our own food in order to provide for our families. Sure, there are still families who rely on a hunter to provide a meat source for the family, and even independent farmers who raise and slaughter their animals to provide food for the family. But more often than not, today's consumer visits a supermarket to provide everything needed to prepare a meal for their family.

As part of the evolutionary process, man has also gotten away from eating a diet of mostly animals and plants. With modern technology, we've embraced other food sources such as sugar(s) and starches found in grains and potatoes. Unfortunately, although times have changed the products that are available for us to consume, our bodies have not made the transition to the same degree. In fact, the human body finds it quite difficult to digest high amounts of carbohydrates derived from starches and diets containing refined sugars. So what is recommended, you ask?

Carbohydrates:

When we wake up in the morning we tend to choose carbohydrates for breakfast, like toast or other items such as breads, biscuits, muffins, cereals, pancakes, or waffles, and foods I consider more snack-like than life-sustaining. Our society tends to eat a diet that contains foods like pasta, corn (which is a grain, not a vegetable), rice, potatoes, and processed foods so many in number that I wouldn't dare try to put a number on it.

The sad thing is that these processed foods are nothing more than processed grains, which are prepared in such a way that we find it difficult to deny ourselves. You know what I'm talking about… the beautiful pastries that call out our names when we attempt to walk by the bakery counter at the store; the delectable breads fresh from the oven that whisper sweet nothings in our ears; or cereals that contain nothing more than sugar, but which we convince ourselves will help reduce cholesterol because marketing tells us so. The fact is these types of products have resulted in higher than normal cholesterol levels, obesity, and chronic diseases such as heart disease in countless Americans.

Obviously, people want and need their carbohydrates. But, we can all live with less of them in our lives and be much more healthy if we limit them. The truth is, our bodies need carbohydrates, we just don't need the number that we consume. When we over-consume them, our bodies are unable to process them in a timely manner and begin storing them as fat. So if your goal is to lose weight, the last thing that you'll want to do is eat something that your body physiologically cannot process.

The key to eating carbohydrates is to pay special attention to your metabolic type and eat healthy foods accordingly. Fruits and vegetables are carbohydrates and we've been led to believe that THESE are the types of foods that our bodies need in order to thrive. While this may be true for some metabolic types, it isn't true for all of them. An example of this would be a Protein Type, who needs carbohydrates, but who should eat carbs belonging to above-ground vegetables and shouldn't include an overabundance of fruits; whereas a Carbohydrates Type can consume root vegetables and grains and get away with it.

An important fact to remember when eating carbohydrates is that once consumed, these foods will elevate blood glucose (sugar). While this may not sound serious, it can be, as the pancreas then responds to the increase in sugar by releasing insulin into the bloodstream, which will lower the body's glucose levels. Sounds harmless – right? Well, expanded upon further, you might want to know that insulin is a hormone that will result in the body storing excess carbohydrate calories as fat in the thighs, abdomen, and buttocks. This is because insulin treats the rise in glucose as a sign of impending famine. Additionally, the production of insulin will often trigger the suppression of other important hormones: glucagon and human growth hormone, which are responsible for the burning of fat and the promotion of healthy muscle development in the body.

If you're going to eat a diet rich in carbohydrates, and you want to be successful at healthy weight loss, you'll want to determine the right quantity of carbohydrates that your body can process for fuel and energy for the day (to avoid their storage in fat cells), and consume the right types of carbohydrates to alleviate feelings of hunger (to prevent you from snacking after you've consumed a meal).

Bread:

I love to bake it and I'm guilty of over-eating it, like most Americans. Known to be the most consumed and most popular carbohydrate to mankind, the negative effects are alarming.

Although there are many types of bread: White, Rye, Pumpernickel, Whole Grain, Whole Wheat, Rice, Oat, and even cornbread, the only bread that is recommended for healthy weight-loss is Ezekiel 4:9. Why? Ezekiel 4:9 is bread made from freshly sprouted organically-grown grains. It is naturally flavorful, meaning that it doesn't need extra ingredients spread onto it to make it taste better, and it is loaded with nutrients. This bread is rich in protein. In fact, through the combination of the six grains and legumes (wheat, barley, beans, lentils, millet, and spelt) a complete protein is created that closely parallels the protein found in organic milk and eggs. The end result is bread that contains 84.3% as much protein as the highest recognized source of protein containing all 9 of the essential amino acids. In fact, there are 18 different amino acids contained within this bread, all from vegetable sources, and it contains all the vitamins, minerals, and natural fiber that a person needs. And best of all – there is no added fat.

Okay, there is one more "best of all." Ezekiel bread is the perfect solution for individuals who suffer with indigestion. With a little explanation, here's why.

Sprouting, as in soaking the grains in water and allowing them to germinate, causes a number of biochemical reactions in the grain which provide multiple benefits: it increases the amount of healthy nutrients and reduces the amount of harmful anti-nutrients. This sprouting process may result in an increase in vital nutrients. Some studies indicate that by sprouting grains it increases the amino acid lysine.

Plants contain a limited amount of amino acids, so through the process of sprouting it increases the efficiency that the proteins in the grain has and can be used for both structural and functional purposes in the human body. Also, the combination of grains with legumes may increase the protein quality to a degree. It has been suggested in multiple studies that sprouting the wheat may actually lead to significant increases in soluble fiber, folate, Vitamins C and E, and Beta-Carotene. Because the sprouting process also breaks down the starch, which takes place as the seed uses energy to fuel sprouting, sprouted grains may have slightly less carbohydrates. Great for those of you counting carbs!

Through the sprouting process you are left with grains that have lower amounts of anti-nutrients or substances that inhibit the absorption of nutrients such as minerals like:

- Phytic Acid is a substance found in grains and many other foods. It can bind minerals like Zinc, Calcium, Magnesium and Iron and prevent them from being absorbed. Sprouting modestly reduces phytic acid.

- Enzyme inhibitors are present in seeds, which protect them from spontaneously germinating but may also make the nutrients in them harder to access. Sprouting inactivates some of them.

Another benefit of sprouting is that it reduces the amount of gluten, a protein that many people are sensitive to and is found in wheat, spelt, rye and barley. What this means in layman's terms:

Due to the reduction in anti-nutrients, Ezekiel bread may be easier to digest and the nutrients in it are more accessible to the body.

Consumers have been long led to believe that whole wheat bread is the way to go. The problem is that it contains processed wheat, which is deficient in nutrients and results in an overabundance of digestive disorders such as irritable bowel syndrome and constipation.

Note: If you are committed to a diet free of gluten, you will be intolerant of Ezekiel 4:9.

For those of you interested in preparing your own Ezekiel bread, I've included the recipe in the back of this book.

Glycemic Index:

If you're familiar with Weight Watchers and various other weight-loss programs, or if you're diabetic, you'll undoubtedly have heard the term "glycemic index" when referring to the manner in which you should combine the foods you eat for optimum results. The GI (Glycemic Index) has determined what foods convert to sugar and at what rate. It is used to figure out how quickly a food will affect the blood sugar so that you can eat foods that will help to maintain balance and not trigger a rapid release of insulin, which we know will trigger the body to store fat.

When attempting to lose weight, actual loss of fat vs. water weight will be accomplished more easily if you choose low-GI carbohydrates: vegetables and some, but not all, fruits. You'll also want to consider certain grains and beans and make it a goal to avoid high-GI foods altogether.

Salt:

With high blood pressure on the rise, everyone should consider a diet low in sodium. Why? Because most Americans consume the wrong kind of salt - table salt or commercially processed salt. Contrary to popular belief, the human body needs salt for several of the body's normal functions, so eliminating it entirely wouldn't make sense. What does make sense is using salt that actually provides your system with what it needs and eliminating from your diet what it doesn't.

Unrefined sea salt is the type of salt that the body needs. It provides the sodium that is an essential nutrient that the body cannot produce itself and is necessary for sustaining life. Plus, it provides chloride, which is required for preserving the acid-base balance within the body, aiding the absorption of potassium, supplying the stomach with the digestive acid it must have, and enhances the ability of the blood to carry carbon dioxide from respiring tissues to the lungs.

Research has been conducted in the United States on both commercially produced salt and on sea salt. The findings on sea salt have been published in French, German, and Portuguese, so unfortunately for Americans, the truth about this type of salt vs. table salt is yet to be discovered and shared with medical patients. As a result, our doctors often suggest that people should avoid salt altogether. Well, based on what we know about the human body's basic need for salt, this is bad advice. Better advice would be to simply use the right kind of salt – sea salt.

Refined white table salt, which is in most of the pantries across America, is different from unrefined sea salt, and therefore the way it affects the human body is not the same. White table salt is made of isolated synthetic sodium chloride (from typical refined salt), which contains none of the minerals and trace elements that unrefined sea salt does, so the body treats it as a poison. It also contains anti-caking agents, which are aluminum based. If you aren't aware of the dangers of aluminum, it has been linked with heavy metal toxicity and possibly Alzheimer's disease. Additionally, other illnesses and disorders have been linked to ingredients in table salt, including sodium silicoaluminate, which is thought to be associated with kidney problems and mineral malabsorption, and sodium acetate, used as a preservative, which may cause elevated blood pressure, kidney disturbances, and water retention. (Chek 2004, 78).

Sodium is important in your quest to lose weight. So instead of eliminating the product from your diet, simply switch to a product that actually is needed by your body for optimal functioning. Celtic sea salt is a good choice and can be found in many health food stores. It is very healthy for the human body and elicits the opposite response from the body. It contains 90 trace elements provided by Mother Nature in the Earth's crust, which leads to its grayish color, plus it is moist, which maintains the salt and minerals in a form that the body can assimilate. Best of all, patients with high blood pressure can use it and benefit, but only if they eliminate all forms of processed salt, sodium, and table salt from their diets.

Note: For athletes, adding a pinch of Celtic sea salt to each liter of bottled water consumed will provide and maintain electrolytes and energy levels necessary for performance.

Soy:

By now you probably know how I feel about cow's milk. If you don't remember, you should probably review the section about Dairy Products again, because although I think I was pretty clear on the subject, maybe you were having a lull in your focus, or the doorbell rang, or perhaps your favorite song was being played. Whatever your particular situation, take a moment to review the section again before moving forward.

Since I don't consume cow's milk, you may be asking yourself what I drink instead. Most people who ask the question assume that I've replaced it with soymilk. That is not the case. I don't believe soy to be the miracle product that others believe it to be. In fact, vegetarians have chosen soy to replace meat products in their diets over the years, only to wind up with serious reproductive disorders and hypothyroidism (Daniel 2005).

Let me provide you with a little history on the subject. The soybean is an oil-laden Asian legume that grows in pods. Its original purpose was to fertilize the soil in between crops in order to provide richer soils. Consumption of the soybean often led to digestive discomforts in humans. Therefore, it wasn't consumed as a regular staple – until fermentation was discovered.

In the United States, soy products are served unfermented, which means that the anti-nutrients that are deactivated by fermentation are still active. Additionally, the unfermented products are processed, which results in their proteins becoming impure, which increases the amount of carcinogens (Daniel 2005, 156).

Soy-based Food Products:

In the United States, soy has been used for many different food products, including tofu, soybean oil (used to feed animals such as poultry and farmed fish), soy milk, protein powders, soy sausages, soy burgers, energy bars, veggie burgers, low-carbohydrate pastas, soy chili, soy patties made to taste and resemble chicken patties, and many foods which contain either soy protein isolate, or soy protein concentrate and texturized vegetable protein. Unfortunately, due to technological advances in food processing services, we've managed to produce the most unhealthy modern soy food products in the United States.

Soy Isoflavones:

Why are soy products so unhealthy? Soy products contain plant-derived estrogens (phytoestrogen), which are referred to isoflavones. In studies conducted, they have been shown to decrease the testosterone levels of rats, monkey, and other animals – including humans.

"How is this possible?" you might be asking yourself. The consumption of soy products by adults can disrupt the body's normal/natural hormone levels, altering the reproductive system in both men and women. In women we're talking about increased cramping during menstruation, a heavier flow, and infertility. Men suffer with a decreased libido and lower sperm count. To make matters worse, soy formula is often fed to infants and young children as an alternative to cow's milk. What scientists at the Swiss Federal Health Service have discovered is that infants are very susceptible to soy, in that with each serving of formula, they consume the equivalent of estrogen found in three to five birth control pills (Daniel 2005, 331). This is substantial and can affect a child's overall health and development.

What does this mean for the child's future development? Scientists believe that with the amount of estrogen consumed by children, their future physical maturation and development can be impacted substantially – for boys it could mean delayed puberty and emasculated boys with breasts and undersized penises. For girls, they see early-onset puberty and reproductive problems as they mature.

Finally, the effects on the thyroid are something that you'll want to consider. Adults and children who've consumed large amounts of soy products in any form often complain of fatigue, low energy, depression, hair loss, weight gain, a diminished sex drive, and blemished skin. These symptoms have often been associated with a low-functioning thyroid (Daniel 2005, 329). In most instances, when tested for hypothyroidism, the test results proved positive.

Sweeteners:

This is an area that really steams my bean. With all the hype and advertising campaigns out there, it's no wonder consumers are so confused about what's safe and what's not. So let me take the mystery out of how we sweeten our foods.

Sugar:

Obviously we all know what sugar is, and most of us know from what it is derived. But did you know that Americans eat as much as 295 pounds of the sweet substance a year? This is alarming and contributes substantially to the over 60% of the U. S. population that struggles with being overweight or obese. (Chek 2004, 75).

I'm sure that you probably know someone who has Type 2 Diabetes. If you don't, that's fantastic. If you do, you might be surprised to know that sugar is a major player responsible for its onset, along with a diet full of carbohydrates.

Sugar is added to almost every product on the market. Think about your pantry and the items contained therein. I'll bet you've got cereals, cookies, cake mixes, and an entire shelf dedicated to processed foods. If it's processed, it's got sugar in it. The sugar contained in those products, when consumed, actually acts like a poison in the body. When your body ingests sugar, it becomes acidic, requiring that the body pull minerals from the body's tissues to counteract and try to re-establish balance. If you don't understand what this means, it is best described as the body pulling calcium from bones and teeth in order to maintain the necessary balance, which leaves the bones weakened and the teeth susceptible to cavities.

Not only is sugar delicious, it is dangerous. Sugar has been linked to other diseases beside diabetes. It's been attributed to cardiovascular disease and cancer. When too much sugar is introduced to the body, the liver will process as much as it can. What it cannot process, it will store in fat cells or return to the blood in the form of fatty acids. These fatty acids will be transported through the body and deposited among our vital organs, such as the heart, liver, and kidneys, and inactive areas of the body like our stomachs, buttocks, breasts, and thighs. Now, many of you probably don't know that cancer cells can only survive in environments that are incredibly acidic, which means that people who consume large amounts of sugar will be more likely to develop cancer at some point in time. So, it stands to reason that if you consume less sugar and maintain a non-acidic environment, your chances of developing cancer will be less.

You might be asking yourself why the American population is so unaware of these hidden dangers. Marketing, advertising, and lobbying in legislature by industries with really deep products make sugar sound like it is the greatest product of all times and that we can't live without it. Truth is, sugar is in most everything and it comes in many different forms. For instance, you'll ingest close to 20 teaspoons of sugar in a day, although it will be listed on labels under many different names. Walk to your pantry and pick up a container of lemonade, a package of cookies, or even pre-packaged chips. You'll more than likely find one, if not two or three of sugar's alternative names, such as sucrose, maltose, dextrose, and glucose. Added together, you'll immediately understand why the product is sugar laden.

Fruit also contains sugar, but it is in its natural form – fructose. This form of sugar will actually take its time when breaking down within the body. Because of this, both blood sugar and insulin levels remain more balanced. Fructose also results in less stress to the body than sucrose, which is comprised of glucose and fructose. If you'll recall, sucrose results in a sudden "spike" in insulin levels – this is extremely stressful to the body.

Lastly, we want to talk about fruit juice. This is an area where I'll warn you, "Buyer Beware." Fruit juices are very often loaded with sugar. Even though the label may say "fresh juice," what you're probably looking at is a product made from "concentrate," which is the equivalent of "syrup."

Artificial Sweeteners:

This is probably the most offensive group of products on the market when it comes to health and wellness, so I'm going to really focus on this area. I am one of the many Americans who are allergic to them. I actually have a reaction similar to individuals reacting to shellfish allergies. Problem is, artificial sweeteners are found in many different products on the market, from cookies to juice drinks to salad dressings. It's unbelievable when you've learned to read labels and can identify these products. But problems with artificial sweeteners aren't just about allergic reactions, but also about how toxic they can be to your body.

Let's talk about artificial sweeteners and the illnesses associated with each of them.

Alarming research and evidence has been released regarding sweeteners, which have been linked to poisoning people who consume the different artificial sweeteners found in soft drinks and various food products.

Most of you are probably familiar with aspartame, which is frequently used as a sweetener in diet sodas or products that specify "Sugar Free." Aspartame is found on the labels as NutraSweet, Equal, and Spoonful. It is deadly and should be avoided at all costs. The information was brought to light after a young lady was misdiagnosed with Multiple Sclerosis (MS). After being confined to a wheelchair, as she could no longer walk, and having problems with her vision, her problems disappeared when her illness was linked to aspartame poisoning. After taking one pill for aspartame poisoning she was symptom-free.

The overwhelming increase in the number of individuals being diagnosed with both multiple sclerosis and systemic lupus has been linked to various toxins that we consume in our everyday diets - most notably - aspartame. Let me explain how aspartame affects our system.

The Dangers of Aspartame:

The wood alcohol that is found in aspartame, when the temperature of the product containing the ingredient exceeds 86 degrees Fahrenheit, converts to formaldehyde and then becomes formic acid, which leads to metabolic acidosis. Formic acid is the poison found in fire ant stings. The methanol toxicity mimics the symptoms of multiple sclerosis and systemic lupus, among other illnesses. Due to the undetectable mimicry, individuals are misdiagnosed repeatedly with the above illnesses, and unfortunately are then treated incorrectly. Multiple sclerosis is not a death sentence, as we've seen Jerry Lewis live with the illness for more than 20 years, but methanol toxicity is!!!

Systemic lupus, which is almost as prominent as MS these days, has been linked to drinkers of Diet Coke and Diet Pepsi. The problem is that individuals who've been diagnosed with the illness do not know that their condition has been linked to aspartame and continue to enjoy the beverages containing the ingredient, which may lead to a life-threatening condition, as the continued use will irritate the lupus.

Aspartame Linked to the Following Illnesses:

It is quite possible that you may suffer from illnesses that have been linked to aspartame poisoning. For example, individuals with systemic lupus became asymptotic after eliminating diet sodas from their daily diet. Equally as impressive was the number of individuals diagnosed with multiple sclerosis who saw a reduction in their symptoms once they quit consuming aspartame/diet drinks.

There are other illnesses that have been linked to the over-consumption of aspartame including:

- Fibromyalgia
- Muscle spasms
- Numbness in the Legs
- Cramps
- Vertigo
- Dizziness
- Headaches
- Tinnitus
- Joint Pain
- Unexplainable depression
- Anxiety attacks
- Slurred speech
- Blurred vision
- Memory loss

These illness or symptoms are linked to aspartame poisoning. The good news is, often these illnesses or symptoms can be reversed by simply eliminating this ingredient from your diet.

Information on Diet Soda: News Flash!!!

I'll bet you didn't know that diet sodas are NOT a diet product! In fact, diet drinks are chemically altered multiple sodium (salt) and aspartame containing products that result in individuals craving carbohydrates. By consuming these products regularly, you are more likely to gain weight than to lose it. These products also contain formaldehyde, which stores in fat cells, often around the hips and thighs. If you're familiar with formaldehyde, you know that it is a toxin that has been linked to cancer and is used in the preservation of tissue specimens. Recognizing this detail, why would you want to introduce it to your body? Dr. H. J. Roberts stated that by eliminating diet products from his patient's consumption habits, they lost an average of 19 pounds over the trial period.

Diabetics and Aspartame:

Believe it or not, aspartame is dangerous for individuals diagnosed with diabetes. This is particularly vital information for me, in that my father died after slipping into a diabetic coma. He lived on diet sodas, which he kept in cases behind the driver's seat of his vehicle. This inevitably increased the product temperature in excess of 86 degrees Fahrenheit, thereby exposing him to the dangers associated with metabolic acidosis.

Aspartame increases the blood sugar in diabetics, thus many diabetics suffer acute memory loss due to the aspartic acid and phenylalanine, which become neurotoxic when taken without the other amino acids necessary for proper insulin-sugar balance. Unfortunately, I learned this information when it was too late for my father. I want to share a little more on this topic.

When a diabetic consumes aspartame, it passes the blood/brain barrier, which then deteriorates the neurons of the brain. This deterioration causes various levels of brain damage and can result in seizures, depression, manic depression, panic attacks, and uncontrollable anger and rage. These symptoms are NOT limited to diabetics and can be found in non-diabetics as well.

If you or someone that you know is diabetic or prefers beverages and other ingredients that are dietary in nature WITHOUT the aspartame, there are other naturally derived sugars that can be used, however, checking with your physician is always recommended before switching products.

- Nature's Hollow Tastes Like Honey
- Joseph's Maltitol Sweetener
- Truvia
- SweetLeaf Sweetener All Natural SteviaPlus
- Xlear, Inc. XyloSweet
- PureVia

In addition to **Stevia,** there are other natural sweeteners that are used by diabetics and persons eating a low carbohydrate diet. Such sweeteners include:

- Lo Han Fruit Extract – SlimSweet, SugarNot
- Agave Nectar & Syrup
- Yacon Syrup (Molasses-like taste)
- Xylitol Gum or Xylitol Gum
- Just Like Sugar

For individuals who MUST have their sodas, Zevia brand, which can be purchased at many local health food or natural food stores, is a suitable alternative to diet sodas. Again, check with your health care professional.

There is more to learn about artificial sweeteners that I simply must share with you, as there truly are so many misconceptions about how "this" product is healthier than "that" one. I cannot move forward without providing you the full picture about how they impact individuals. Before moving forward, let me sum up aspartame for you.

Aspartame is a powerful drug and one that the public NEEDS to be aware of, as it ultimately affects the health and wellness of everyone exposed to the poison. Become an educated consumer!!! Read labels and always choose healthier alternatives, and PLEASE share this article with at least five individuals that you care about. I'm counting you as one of the individuals that I care about.

By now, you can probably see for yourself that all sweeteners are not the same. And after sharing the above information with others, I was immediately bombarded with questions about the other sugars. So here are the answers.

Artificial sweeteners, each one on the market (Sweet 'N Low, Splenda, NutraSweet, the list goes on and on) comes with its own list of health warnings. We've been told that Splenda, another very popular artificial sweetener, is different from all the other artificial sweeteners' past failures. According to the claims, it is the perfect sugar substitute: as sweet as sugar, but no calories; as sweet as sugar, but no surge in insulin; as sweet as sugar, but no side effects or long-term health damage.

Nothing is as sweet as the TRUTH. So here you have it.

A Biochemistry Moment:

Splenda, the trade name for sucralose, is a synthetic compound stumbled upon in 1976 by scientists in Britain seeking a new pesticide formulation. It is true that the Splenda molecule is comprised of sucrose (sugar), but perhaps first and foremost, it is NOT a natural product. It is a chlorinated artificial sweetener. "Sucralose is a disaccharide that is made from sucrose in a five-step process that selectively substitutes three atoms of chlorine for three hydroxyl groups in the sugar molecule. Sucralose is a free-flowing, white crystalline form that is soluble in water and stable both in crystalline form and in most aqueous solutions; it has a sweetness intensity that is 320 to 1,000 times that of sucrose, depending on the food application."

FDA/CFSAN Federal Register 63 FR 16417 April 3, 1998 – Final Rule: Sucralose

Many consumers operate under the belief that simply because a product is approved by the U.S. Food & Drug Administration (FDA), and has made it onto the shelves in retail markets, that it has been thoroughly tested for both short and long-term effects on humans. This is in fact not always the case. According to Duke University, a new study has been underway which has discovered the following details about use of this particular sweetener:

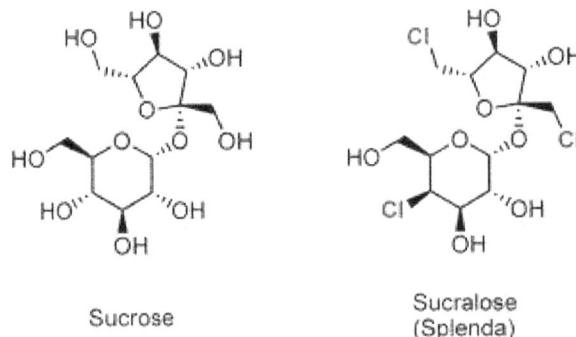

Sucrose

Sucralose
(Splenda)

Splenda "suppresses beneficial bacteria and directly affects the expression of the transporter P-gp and cytochrome P-450 isozymes that are known to interfere with the bioavailability of drugs and nutrients. These findings were discovered in products containing sucralose levels that are approved by the FDA for use in the food supply.

Approved by the Food and Drug Administration and cited by the Mayo Clinic and other gate-keeping health agencies as safe alternatives to sugar, artificial sweeteners such as aspartame (Equal, NutraSweet, NatraTaste), saccharin (Sweet 'N Low, Sugar Twin) and sucralose (Splenda) remain a subject of concern and debate among consumers, health-care professionals, and researchers. Opponents of the sweeteners believe anecdotal evidence links them to a lengthy list of illnesses and symptoms, including headaches, seizures, hyperactivity, cancer, tumors, glandular problems, fatigue, and fibromyalgia."

The Courier Post, Cherry Hill, N.J., August 15, 2004, Shawn Rhea

So, is Splenda Safe? Comparing Apples to Apples....

The truth is that we really don't know yet. The studies conducted haven't been of any suitable duration in which to assess the side effects of Splenda in humans. Manufacturers who've conducted studies have done only short-term studies. Those showed that very high doses of sucralose (far beyond what would be expected in an ordinary diet) resulted in *shrunken thymus glands, enlarged livers, and kidney disorders* in rodents. (A more recent study also shows that Splenda significantly decreases beneficial gut flora, similar to the results found at Duke University.)

Now, here's the doozy... In this case, the FDA decided that because these studies weren't based on human test animals, they were not conclusive. Keep in mind though, that rats had been chosen for the testing specifically because they metabolize sucralose more like humans than any other animal used for testing. Looked at another way, the FDA has attempted to ride the fence — they accepted the manufacturer's studies on rats because the manufacturer had shown that rats and humans metabolize the sweetener in similar ways, but ignored the safety concerns based on the fact that rats and humans are different. You be the judge? Based on my findings, determining whether something is safe (or not) in laboratory rats isn't a definitive answer, as we've seen countless examples of foods and drugs that have been proven dangerous to humans that were first found to be safe in laboratory rats, both in short and long-term studies.

There is evidence surfacing identifying the side effects of Splenda little by little. Sucralose has been identified as a possible trigger for migraine headaches. Other information reported by individuals on adverse reactions to Splenda or sucralose collected by the Sucralose Toxicity Information Center include skin rashes/flushing, panic-like agitation, dizziness and numbness, diarrhea, swelling, muscle aches, headaches, intestinal cramping, bladder issues, and stomach pain. Unfortunately no one can say to what degree consuming Splenda affects the rest of us, and there are no long-term studies in humans with large numbers of subjects to say one way or the other if it's safe for *everyone*.

What's in a name? That which we call Splenda... By any other name would taste as sweet (or sweeter) than sugar:

If this sounds familiar, it should, as we followed the same path with aspartame, the main ingredient in Equal and NutraSweet. Almost all of the independent research studies conducted on aspartame found dangerous side effects in rodents. The FDA chose not to take these findings into account when it approved aspartame for public use. Over the past 15 years, those same side effects increasingly appeared in humans. Not in everyone, of course — but in a significant number of individuals, especially those who were vulnerable to the chemical structure of aspartame.

Artificial sweeteners have been used for decades. Some leave individuals near death while some people don't react as poorly — the problem is, you never know until you or someone that you love and care about is already sick. Scientists have referred to Splenda as a mild mutagen, based on the amount of the sweetener that is absorbed. Right now, it's anyone's guess what portion of the population is being exposed to the dangers of Splenda or already suffering from Splenda side effects.

Until an independent, unbiased research group conducts long-term studies on humans, and I'm not talking about studies similar to the six-month trials currently being considered, how can we be certain? With the vast number of Splenda products being added to the supermarket shelves, it looks as if we are in the process of becoming the guinea pig for another round of public experiments — without our consent and permission, of course. Sadly, we may not know the health implications for decades to come and as with all things, time will ALWAYS tell the truth.

So I urge you to be concerned about the potential dangers of Splenda — as with any unnatural substance you put into your body. And, as you've probably guessed, I am especially concerned about its use for children, which I recommend you avoid at all costs.

Good Old Fashioned Sugar vs. Artificial Sweeteners (Splenda):

As with anything, moderation is key!!! But if you're unable to ingest the "real stuff," what should you do? There are other alternatives available to you, as mentioned above. I believe alternative sweeteners can serve a purpose for some people, but only if they've been tried and found safe for consumption. And that has to do with the old question — which is better, sugar or another form of sweetener? Let's start with sugar and where the problem(s) really begin.

Feeding your sweet tooth with better nutrition by choosing to build snacks and meals from whole foods, which means foods that have not been processed and manipulated, is better for you than any other option. Your food should resemble its source as closely as possible; for instance, fresh fish vs. a fish stick. And this includes sugar. Even if you don't have a reaction or sensitivity to sugar, continue to use refined sugar rarely, if ever. Instead, sweeten sparingly with the more nutritionally complex natural sugars such as honey, rice syrup, molasses, and maple syrup.

Now, if you already suffer from weight gain, diabetes, inflammation, chronic pain, migraines, headaches, or depression, you may have what's known as sugar intolerance. Check with your healthcare provider and try the elimination diet. This simply means eliminating sugar entirely from your diet for a couple of weeks, then reintroducing it for a day to see how you feel. Many people are amazed at how much better they feel after breaking the sugar habit.

Tips for a Healthier You:

If you'll remember a few very simple healthy habits, you can consume sugar, the real deal, without the complications. Here are a few tips to help:

- **Take a daily multivitamin to support your body's nutritional needs.**

- **Eat protein, healthy fats, and complex carbohydrates for breakfast.** Simple carbs and sugar can "fire up" your insulin receptors and spark those crazy sugar cravings. Starting your day with a sugary or high-carb breakfast dooms you to a day of up-and-down blood sugar levels, which will drive you to eat too much of the wrong things all day long.

- **Shop the perimeter of your grocery store.** Avoid the processed foods in the center aisles. Read all labels and be cautious of food that contains aspartame, neotame, saccharin, acesulfame K, or sucralose. No studies have been done on the safety of mixing artificial sweeteners, and who wants to become a guinea pig to find out? So if you consume them, do so prudently.

- **Minimize or avoid products that have sugar, high-fructose corn syrup, or corn syrup near the top of their ingredient list.** Sugar can also be disguised as evaporated cane juice, cane sugar, beet sugar, glucose, sucrose, maltose, maltodextrin, dextrose, sorbitol, fructose, corn sugar, fruit juice concentrate, barley malt, caramel, and carob syrup.

- **Keep a bowl of fresh ripe fruit nearby to snack on,** to relieve your sugar cravings. Think primitive and eat fruit that is in season. The fresher the fruit, the more succulent and satisfying it will be. You may find you don't need anything sweeter!

- **If you are craving something sweet, don't feel guilty.** We're often made to feel that avoiding sugar is only matter of willpower, but it's more complicated than that. Most of the time, uncontrollable or patterned cravings stem from a malfunctioning metabolism or low serotonin. Work on healthy nutrition and you'll find your cravings will disappear.

- **Indulge yourself from time to time.** Remember, we have sweet taste buds for a reason. Try a piece of fruit first — you may find your cravings diminish. If you still want a piece of chocolate or pie, go ahead! But savor it slowly, like a rare treat you may not have again for a while. Once your brain is allowed to fully register the experience, you may find your cravings are subdued after only a few bites. And, to help balance out the accompanying insulin surge, eat a piece of protein with it. Just make it a treat, not a habit.

- **Remember that wine and alcohol are sugar.** When it comes to sugar, having a glass or two of wine every day is just like a daily dessert. Sip smart!

- **If you feel the sugar urge coming on**, first take a short walk after eating and breathe in deeply. It's likely you won't want dessert after all! And if you do, you'll appreciate it more.

- **Focus more on what you'd like to cook and eat than what you shouldn't.** If you listen to your body, it may surprise you with a craving for eggs, not a diet soda.

With these "smart tips," you may be surprised at how you can safely manage your eating and consumption habits to exclude the need for sugar-laden foods. Managing your appetite may make all the difference in the world in your desire for consuming something sweet.

Stevia:

Stevia was briefly mentioned above as a healthy alternative to sugar and artificial sweeteners. It is an herb, which is incredibly sweet when compared to sugar. It is also a calorie-free food and perfect for people who are watching their weight. It doesn't trigger an increase in blood sugar, so your body won't send insulin to the rescue. Best of all, Stevia isn't toxic like the other products we've reviewed, and has in fact been used for hundreds of years for beverages and baking.

Being IN CONTROL of your eating habits instead of BEING CONTROLLED is truly the key!!!

Water:

Ask anyone this question, "What beverage should you include in your diet every single day?" and, if they're serious, you'll probably get the same answer. Of course the answer is water. Unfortunately, however, not many people actually live by the advice that they'll provide another human being. Sadly, people do not understand just how vital water is to a healthy nutritional program. However, if you ask, "How many glasses of water should a person consume a day?" they'll all know the answer

– between 8 to 10 glasses. Why is water imperative to losing weight? Let's discover the reason together.

You've heard the saying, "Milk, it does a body good!" Well, in reality, water does a body good, and here's why.

- Water is a natural diuretic. What this means is that individuals who retain fluids need to drink more water. When the body does not get enough water, it becomes threatened and will begin holding onto every drop of water that it can – retention. When you provide the body with the water that it needs, it will begin to release water that is being retained.

- Water is critical to eliminating waste. By now, you've probably discovered that the "junk" the body holds onto in the form of stored fat and toxins will definitely want to be expelled. When losing weight, water consumption will help the body flush these toxins from the body.

- Water is a natural laxative. The human body is somewhat remarkable when it comes to providing the necessary vitamins, minerals, fat, and water that it needs to sustain life. When the body isn't supplied with enough water, it will actually pull water from other sources, like internal organs. If the colon isn't moist, the stool becomes dry and can be difficult to pass. This is often felt and described as constipation. Often, gas, bloating, and painful elimination will result. Drinking enough water will help keep the body hydrated, resulting in proper bowel functions and elimination.

- Water is a natural appetite suppressant. Forget the pills and gimmicks that encourage you to drink this, take that, or sprinkle your food… by simply drinking eight ounces of water fifteen minutes before a meal, you'll be more likely to eat less and also be able to determine if you're actually hungry OR thirsty.

- Water is necessary for the body to metabolize stored fat. Without water, the kidneys cannot function properly. If the kidneys aren't working the way they are intended, they have to rely on reinforcement, such as the liver, to help do their job. Adequate and proper liver function is necessary for the body to lose weight, and if it isn't able to complete its role in metabolizing fat due to it providing assistance, more fat will be stored and less lost, resulting in overall weight loss becoming slow and perhaps nonexistent.

Individuals require different amounts of water for proper functioning. A good rule of thumb is to take your weight and divide by two, and then drink that number of ounces each and every day.

Sounds easy, right? Not so much for many individuals who don't like to drink water. I enjoy water and drink it pretty much with every meal. You might be asking yourself, "If I drink tea, does the water content count?" Nope!!! In fact, if you're drinking caffeinated tea, you'll need to drink an extra eight ounces of water to offset the amount of caffeine consumed in other eight-ounce beverages. This is true for coffee, soda, and anything else containing caffeine. You'll also want to drink an extra eight ounces of water if you've exercised.

Some people actually mistake thirst for hunger, as the body interprets both sensations the same. It is recommended that the moment you feel hunger pains rearing their heads, that you immediately drink water. Often times, people are simply dehydrated when hunger pains are triggered. By hydrating your body, you may actually satisfy the feelings of hunger (which were actually thirst). In studies that were conducted, individuals who consumed the water after experiencing hunger pains actually lost between 35 – 40 pounds in less than a year's time. (Batmanghelidj 1992, 99).

In the movie *Water Boy*, starring Adam Sandler, you may remember the famous line, "Now that's good quality H2O." Drinking high quality water is important if you're hoping to benefit from the water consumed. Water is highly processed these days, and loaded with chemicals and toxins that the body doesn't need. For example, today water is contaminated with heavy metals, chlorine, fluoride, and other toxins that are waterborne. If you elect to use tap water and you're on a well or city water, you'll want to consider purchasing a filtration system that will help to eliminate these additives.

If you choose to buy bottled water, you'll want to do your homework and determine which brands are best. Another consideration is packaging of water. Bottles are best because plastic bottles are known to contain Bisphenol-A, or BPA, which is toxic and can leach into your drinking water if the bottles are frozen or exposed to sunlight. This toxic chemical, when consumed, emulates estrogen in the body, which has been linked to many medical disorders. If you'd like more information on Bisphenol-A, please visit http://childrentopics.com/?p=670

CHAPTER EIGHT
METABOLIC TYPE TEST

This may be the single most important part of this health and wellness guide, in that through determining your metabolic type, you'll be able to customize menus utilizing foods that will ultimately help you lose weight by creating healthy combinations of food.

I have compiled a test that you will want to take after monitoring your dietary habits for a few weeks. You can certainly take the test now, but your answers may not be accurate. I'll show you what I mean. Upon first taking the test, I thought that I was considered a Mixed-Metabolic type. I created a diet based on this information; however, after utilizing the diet for a couple of weeks, I found that I was starving within 20 minutes after consuming a meal. This metabolic type test proved inaccurate as I began monitoring how I felt after eating a different variety of carefully prepared meals based upon metabolic typing. It was after wasting two weeks eating the wrong combination of foods that I discovered that I'm actually a Protein Metabolic Type, which made a tremendous difference in the foods I should have been eating.

Determining your metabolic type is a pretty simple task. You'll simply review the questions below, answering them honestly (not the way that you think they should be answered), as there is no right or wrong answer. Then, you'll tally your answers and be able to decipher the type of metabolism your body actually has.

I'm going to provide (3) different tests for you to use in order to accurately determine your metabolic type.

Metabolic Type Test #1

There are pretty substantial differences between the three, so it's no wonder so many people show no loss when dieting and simply give up! They're eating the wrong stuff!

I would advise everyone **WHO IS NOT HAVING ANY SUCCESS AT LOSING** to read the following excerpt, take a simple test, and find out what **exactly** your body prefers to run on. Trust me; it could make a world of difference in your weight loss efforts!

Winning by Losing

By Jillian Michaels
Metabolic Typing

You may be thinking that as long as you stay within your caloric range for the week, you can eat whatever you want. Although it's true that at a basic level weight loss is simple math, there is more to losing weight and getting healthy than just numbers. As you restrict your caloric intake, it is absolutely essential that you eat the right kinds of food to build muscle, strengthen your immune system, and stay energized throughout the process. Sounds simple, right? It would be, except that the way to do this is different for everyone.

Determining Your Metabolic Type

For many years nutritional science has taken a generic, overly standardized approach to health and weight loss. This is why there is no one diet that works for everyone. There was all that hype about the Atkins diet, but Kelly, one of my contestants on The Biggest Loser, lost just one pound in a month of sticking to Atkins. Because I know that we are all different and need to diet according to our specific body's characteristics, I was able to coach her to lose 55 pounds in three months. We were working together on the show, and she lost 35 more after that.

Why? Inherited genetics make each one of us unique, from the color of our hair right down to the way our organs function. This uniqueness extends to the way our cells convert nutrients into energy. In order to know how to get the most nutritional bang for your calorie buck, you need to understand your unique metabolic type. Once you do, you can begin to custom design your new dietary lifestyle around the foods that will help you achieve and maintain your ideal weight while also optimizing your physical energy, strength, and mental clarity.

Metabolic typing is really just fancy talk for figuring out how your body processes what you eat — more specifically, how your body deals with the three basic macronutrients in food: carbohydrates, proteins, and fats. Imagine that you are a furnace: your body takes the food you eat and burns it with oxygen to convert its caloric content into energy. This process is known as oxidation, and it's how the carb content in your food gets turned into glucose and released into the blood. When glucose is released into the blood, the pancreas is cued to release insulin to "clean" your blood of any sugar that is not being used by the body as energy and carry it to your cells, where it gets stored as fat. The fact that we all oxidize the nutrients in our food in different ways is the reason why a particular diet will work for one person and not for another. If you know more about how the nutrients in your food act on your system, you can avoid a lot of unnecessary pitfalls and really maximize your results as you continue on your journey toward total health.

Although rates can vary a lot from one person to the next, most people can be classified according to three basic groups:

1. Fast oxidizers
2. Slow oxidizers
3. Balanced oxidizers

Fast oxidizers burn through the nutrients in their food very rapidly, with the consequence that the carb content is broken down to glucose and released into the blood almost at once. This sudden increase in blood sugar triggers a rapid release of large amounts of insulin to clean away excess sugar, which is stored as fat in your cells. The more carb content in your food, the more energy will be available to your body right away, and the greater the chance that it will not be needed and get stored as fat. Insulin is a quick and effective blood-cleanser, and the dramatic leaps and falls in blood sugar levels that result from fast oxidation lead to the sugar crash effect. For a fast oxidizer, foods with high carb ratios cause fatigue and carb cravings as well as promote fat storage.

Fast oxidizers should eat foods with more proteins and fats in order to slow down their rate of oxidation and insulin release and to better promote stable blood sugar and sustained energy levels.

Slow oxidizers burn through the nutrients in their food slowly and do not release the glucose from carbohydrates into the blood quickly enough, which means that they do not get converted into glucose, and energy production and availability are delayed.

A slow oxidizer should eat foods with higher ratios of carbs, since protein and fat slow the rate of oxidation and energy production even further.

Balanced oxidizers fall right in between the two. They require foods that have equal quantities of protein, fat, and carbs in order to optimally process, produce, and use the energy from their food.

Now that we have defined the different metabolic types, you're probably wondering how you're supposed to know what's happening in your blood every time you have a snack. Don't worry — there's a test, and you can take it right now, and all you need is a pencil and paper. The test is made up of a series of detailed questions that bear on everything from the foods you crave to the dryness of your skin. These questions cover such a wide range of physical attributes because scientists now believe that metabolic type, i.e., the way in which your body processes nutrients, is wired right into a part of your central nervous system that controls a host of other functions within your body. Consequently, if you take a closer look at some of the peripheral functions in your own body, they will shed light on your particular oxidative type and help you pinpoint your specific nutritional needs.

Oxidizer Test

For each of these questions, circle the response that best applies to you. You may not know the answer right off the bat — it may take a couple of days if you have to see a pattern - but really think about these questions and analyze how different foods affect your body and your moods. The better you know yourself, the greater your odds of achieving exactly the results you want.

In the morning, you:

A. Don't eat breakfast.

B. Have something light like fruit, toast, or cereal.

C. Have something heavy like eggs, bacon or steak, and hash browns.

At a buffet, the foods you choose are:

A. Light meats like fish and chicken, vegetables and salad, a sampling of different desserts.

B. A mixture of A and C.

C. Heavy, fatty foods like steak, ribs, pork chops, cheeses, and cream sauces.

Your appetite at lunch is:

A. Low.

B. Normal.

C. Strong.

Your appetite at dinner is:

A. Low.

B. Normal.

C. Strong.

Caffeine makes you feel:

A. Great—it helps you focus.

B. Neutral—you can take it or leave it.

C. Jittery or nauseous.

The types of foods you crave are (sugar is not listed because everyone craves sugar when they are tired or run-down):

A. Fruits, bread, and crackers.

B. Both A and C.

C. Salty foods, cheeses, and meats.

For dinner, you prefer:

A. Chicken or fish, salad, and rice.

B. No preference—choice varies daily.

C. Heavier, fatty foods like pastas, steak, and potatoes.

After dinner, you:

A. Need to have something sweet.

B. Could take dessert or leave it.

C. Don't care for sweets and would rather have something salty like popcorn.

The types of sweets you like are:

A. Sugary candies.

B. No preference.

C. Ice cream or cheesecake.

Eating fatty foods like meat and cheese before bed:

A. Interferes with your sleep.

B. Doesn't bother you.

C. Improves your sleep.

Eating carbs like breads and crackers before your bed:

A. interferes with your sleep, but they're better than heavier foods.

B. Doesn't affect you.

C. Is better than nothing, but you sleep better with heavier foods.

Eating sweets before bed:

A. Doesn't keep you from sleeping at all.

B. Sometimes makes you feel restless in bed.

C. Keeps you up all night.

Each day, you eat:

A. Two or three meals with no snacks.

B. Three meals with maybe one light snack.

C. Three meals and a lot of snacks.

Your attitude toward food is:

A. You often forget to eat.

B. You enjoy food and rarely miss a meal.

C. You love food and it's a central part of your life.

When you skip meals, you feel:

A. Fine.

B. You don't function at your best, but it doesn't really bother you.

C. Shaky, irritable, weak, and tired.

Your attitude toward fatty foods is:

A. You don't like them.

B. You like them occasionally.

C. You crave them regularly.

When you eat fruit salad for breakfast or lunch, you feel:

A. Satisfied.

B. Okay, but you usually need a snack in between meals.

C. Unsatisfied and still hungry.

What kind of food drains your energy?

A. Fatty foods.

B. No food affects you this way.

C. Fruit, candy, or confections, which give you a quick boost, then an energy crash.

Your food portions are:

A. Small—less than average.

B. Average—not more or less than other people.

C. Large—usually more than most people.

How do you feel about potatoes?

A. You don't care for them.

B. You could take them or leave them.

C. You love them.

Red meat makes you feel:

A. Tired.

B. No particular feeling one way or the other.

C. Strong.

A salad for lunch makes you feel:

A. Energized and healthy.

B. Fine, but it isn't the best type of food for you.

C. Sleepy.

How do you feel about salt?

A. Foods often taste too salty.

B. You don't notice one way or the other.

C. You crave salt and salt your food regularly.

How do you feel about snacks?

A. You don't really snack, but you like something sweet if you do.

B. You can snack on anything.

C. You need snacks but prefer meats, cheeses, eggs, or nuts.

How do you feel about sour foods like pickles, lemon juice, or vinegar?

A. You don't like them.

B. They don't bother you one way or the other.

C. You like them.

How do you feel about sweets?

A. Sweets alone can satisfy your appetite.

B. They don't bother you but don't totally satisfy you.

C. You don't feel satisfied and often crave more sweets.

When you just eat meat (bacon, sausage, ham) for breakfast, you feel:

A. Sleepy, lethargic, or irritable.

B. It varies day to day.

C. Full until lunch.

When you eat heavy or fatty foods, you feel:

A. Irritable.

B. Neutral—they don't affect you.

C. Satisfied.

When you feel anxious:

A. Fruits or vegetables calm you down.

B. Eating anything calms you down.

C. Fatty foods calm you down.

You concentrate best when you eat:

A. Fruits and grains.

B. Nothing in particular.

C. Meat and fatty food.

You feel more depressed when you eat:

A. Fatty or heavy foods.

B. Nothing in particular.

C. Fruits, breads, or sweets.

You notice you gain weight when you eat:

A. Fatty foods.

B. No particular food. You gain weight when you overeat.

C. Fruits or carbs.

What type of insomnia, if any, applies to you?

A. You rarely get insomnia from hunger.

B. You rarely get insomnia, but if you do, you often need to eat something in order to fall back asleep.

C. You often wake up during the night and need to eat. If you eat right before bed, it alleviates the insomnia.

Your personality type is:

A. Aloof, withdrawn, or introverted.

B. Neither introverted nor extroverted.

C. Extroverted.

Your mental and physical stamina are better when you eat:

A. Light proteins like egg whites, chicken, or fish and fruits.

B. Any wholesome food.

C. Fatty foods.

Your climate preference is:

A. Warm or hot weather.

B. Doesn't matter.

C. Cold weather.

You have problems with coughing or chest pressure:
If yes, "C"; if no, move on to the next question.

You have a tendency to get cracked skin or dandruff:
If yes, "C"; if no, move on to the next question.

You have a tendency to get light-headed or dizzy:
If yes, "C"; if no, move on to the next question.

Your eyes tend to be:
A. Dry.
B. Fine.
C. Teary.

Your facial coloring is:
A. Noticeably pale.
B. Average.
C. Pink or often flushed.

Your fingernails are:
A. Thick.
B. Average.
C. Thin.

Your gag reflex is:
A. Insensitive.
B. Normal.
C. Sensitive.

You get goose bumps:

A. Often.

B. Occasionally.

C. Very rarely.

You are prone to:

A. Constipation.

B. No stomach problems.

C. Diarrhea.

When insects bite you, your reaction is:

A. Mild.

B. Average.

C. Strong.

Your body type is:

A. Short and stocky.

B. Average.

C. Tall and thin.

Your nose is:

A. Dry.

B. Normal.

C. Runny.

Scoring Your Metabolic Typing Test

When you have finished the test, add up the number of A answers, B answers, and C answers you have circled.

A_____ B_____ C_____

If your number of C answers is 5 or more higher than your number of A or B answers, you are a fast oxidizer.

If your number of A answers is 5 or more higher than your number of B or C answers, you are a slow oxidizer.

If your number of B answers is 5 or more higher than your number of A or C answers, or if neither A, B, nor C's are 5 or more higher than the other two, you are a balanced oxidizer.

If you've answered this questionnaire and you are still not clear which category is the right one for you, there are two other tests you can take to help clarify your metabolic type. These tests are a little drastic and provocative, and they are only intended for those who truly cannot type themselves using the questionnaire.

1. Niacin test: Take 50 milligrams of niacin on an empty stomach. If you experience an immediate flush, you are most likely a fast oxidizer. If you experience a moderate flushing effect, you are a balanced oxidizer. If you experience a significantly delayed flushing or nothing at all, you are a slow oxidizer.

2. Vitamin C test: Take 8 grams of vitamin C in equally divided doses over 8 hours. The fast oxidizer will respond by feeling acidic and uncomfortable, and may even experience other symptoms such as diarrhea, nausea, or increased intestinal gas. A true balanced oxidizer may find that his or her stomach feels less acidic. A slow oxidizer will have no response at all. I'm assuming you have now identified yourself somewhere along the fast-slow continuum. Now it's time to get to know more about your type. Read whichever section applies to you to learn the particular foods and eating habits that are right for your type. If you're good to your metabolism, it'll return the favor by working to help you maintain weight loss and good health.

Fast Oxidizers

You require foods with higher percentages of protein and fat than carbohydrates. Make sure there is protein in everything you eat, including snacks. Your ideal macronutrient ratio is 20 percent carbs, 50 percent protein, 30 percent fat.

Proteins

All proteins are not created equal. The ones that are best for you are high-purine proteins, which are commonly found in fattier meats. This is not to say that you should cut out chicken or fish, but you need the heavier proteins most because they help slow down your rate of oxidation.

Choose from this list of proteins when deciding on a meal or snack:

High Purine: organ meats (pâté, liver, etc.), herring, mussels, sardines, anchovies

Moderate Purine: beef, bacon, dark meat chicken, duck, lamb, spareribs, dark meat turkey, veal, wild game, salmon, shellfish (lobster, shrimp, crab), oysters, scallops, octopus, squid, dark tuna

Low Purine: cottage cheese, milk, yogurt, eggs, cheese, white meat chicken, turkey, fish

Carbohydrates

Your metabolism thrives when your carb intake is limited, but there are different kinds of carbs. Some aren't as bad as others. Avoid simple carbs, which convert to sugar quickly in the bloodstream. The carbs you can incorporate into your diet are the complex kind found mostly in non-starchy vegetables. You can choose from these ideal carbs when deciding on a meal or snack.

Low-Starch vegetables: asparagus, cauliflower, celery, mushrooms, spinach

Fruits: avocado, olives, apples, and pears (in limited quantity and never without protein on the side)

Grains: sprouted grain bread only (Ezekiel bread is a well-known brand that is available at supermarkets and health–food stores)

Legumes, tempeh, tofu

Fats
To best support your metabolism, you should be getting roughly 30 percent of your daily caloric intake from natural oils and fats. Choose these ideal fats when deciding on meal or snack preparation.

Nuts/Seeds (listed in order of protein content): walnuts, pumpkin seeds, peanuts, sunflower seeds, sesame seeds, almonds, cashews, Brazil nuts, filberts, pecans, chestnuts, pistachios, coconut, macadamias

Fat/Oils: butter, cream, almond oil, peanut oil, coconut oil, sesame oil, flaxseed oil, sunflower oil, walnut oil

Along with knowing the foods that are ideal for you, it is important to know the foods that are worst for you. You don't always have to eat off the ideal foods list, but the following foods will sabotage your weight-loss efforts.

1. Don't ever eat a meal that is predominantly carbohydrates.

2. Don't drink alcohol. It causes an increase in blood sugar and fat storage, and it will lead to a sugar crash as well as an increased appetite for carbs. If you choose to have a drink, avoid sugary cocktails, beer, and wine. Stick to clear alcohols like vodka or rum with calorie-free mixers like diet or club soda, and you can always just do what I do and drink it all straight.

3. Don't eat carbohydrates that are high on the glycemic load index. The next chapter will tell you everything you need to know about the GLI. For now all you need to know is to stay away from high-GLI foods. It is important for all metabolic types to watch their high-GLI intake, but it is

especially crucial for you. If you should happen to eat high-GLI foods, make sure to combine them with a protein in order to slow down the production and release of blood sugar.

4. Don't drink too much caffeine. It is true that caffeine can be used as a fat burner and a performance enhancer when exercising. This is only effective, however, when the caffeine is taken in pill form in conjunction with aspirin. In the forms of coffee, tea, and soda, caffeine gives you short-term energy, but does so by getting your adrenal glands to dump adrenaline into your blood like it's going out of style. As a result, when the caffeine leaves your system, your adrenal glands will be depleted for a while, which leaves you feeling weak and tired from substandard blood-adrenaline levels. Caffeine also speeds the rate of oxidation, which is the exact opposite of what you want your nutrients to do. Avoid caffeinated beverages whenever possible and keep your overall caffeine consumption to a minimum.

5. Don't overcook your meat. Avoid overcooked animal products, since heat destroys essential amino acids and valuable enzymes.

You will have fewer physical ailments and feel energized if you eat the foods that contain the ideal macronutrient ratios for your metabolic type. However, these foods are all very high in calories. You must remember to keep within your caloric allowance in order to lose weight.

Slow Oxidizers

In order to best serve your metabolism and feel energized both physically and mentally, you require foods with a higher percentage of carbohydrates. Your ideal macronutrient ratio is 60 percent carbs, 25 percent protein, and 15 percent fat.

Proteins

The best proteins for slow oxidizers are low-purine proteins, which are found in leaner meats. It's not that you can never have steak again, but high-purine, high-fat proteins slow down the rate at which you convert nutrients into energy, which is what you're already doing too slowly, so the less the better. In general, you want to stick to this list.

Low Purine: white meat chicken, turkey breast, lean pork, catfish, cod, flounder, perch, sole, trout, white meat tuna, swordfish, low-fat cheese, low-fat cottage cheese, skim milk, low-fat yogurt, egg whites

Carbohydrates

Although your metabolic type is better than the others at processing carbs, you still have to pick and choose carefully. You want to avoid simple carbs, which convert into sugar very quickly in the bloodstream, and choose complex carbs instead. Follow this list of ideal carbohydrates when deciding on a meal or snack.

Vegetables — Low Starch: asparagus, cauliflower, celery, mushrooms, spinach, broccoli, Brussels sprouts, cabbage, collard greens, cucumbers, garlic, kale, leafy greens, onions, peppers, scallions, sprouts, tomatoes, watercress

Vegetables—Moderate: Starch beets, eggplant, jicama, okra, yellow squash, and zucchini

Fruits: apples, berries, cherries, citrus fruits, peaches, pears, apricots, plums, tropical fruits, olives

Grains: barley, brown rice, buckwheat, corn, couscous, kasha, millet, oat, quinoa, rye, spelt

Legumes, tempeh, tofu, (eat sparingly as they are high in purines) beans, peas (should be eaten fresh, never dried)

Fats

You should be on a low-fat diet to keep your metabolism working smoothly. This does not mean no fat — fat is still an essential part of any healthy diet. You should allow 15 percent of your caloric intake to come from fat. You can go over that percentage if you like, but eating foods that are too high in fat content can make you feel lethargic, anxious, and irritable. Choose from this list of fats when cooking a meal or having a snack.

Nuts/Seeds: raw and unsalted only — be very sparing

Fats/Oils: vegetable or nut oils such as almond, coconut, flaxseed, olive, peanut, sunflower, walnut

It's not enough to know the foods that are ideal for you — you also have to learn which foods are worst for you. If you find yourself straying from the list of suggestions, remind yourself of these guidelines.

1. Don't eat foods that are fatty or that contain high-purine proteins, such as organ meats and fish such as herring and sardines. Limit your intake of fats and oils, as they will slow down your ability to convert food into energy even further. Avoid red meat or dark white meats, and stay away from high-fat dairy, nut butters, and avocados.

2. Don't drink alcohol. This is less of a concern for you than for fast oxidizers, but at the end of the day alcohol still increases your blood sugar and inhibits fat metabolism.

3. Don't drink too much caffeine. This too is less of a concern for you than it is for fast oxidizers, but caffeine gives you energy by acting on your adrenal glands, causing them to overproduce and flood your system with adrenaline. When the caffeine's effect has worn off, your adrenals are exhausted and you are left with lower-than-normal levels of adrenaline in your system, which makes you feel tired and sluggish.

4. Don't exceed one serving per meal of simple or starchy carbs like potato, pasta, or rice, and always eat them with a lean protein to help stabilize your blood sugar.

Remember to consume your ideal foods in accordance with your caloric allowance; otherwise, you will not lose weight.

Balanced Oxidizers

If you are a balanced oxidizer, your diet is the easiest to follow, since you require an equal percentage of carbs, fats, and proteins. You feel at your best on a diet that incorporates a wide range of foods. Your ideal macronutrient ratio is 40 percent carbs, 30 percent protein, and 30 percent fat.

Proteins

You operate best when you are getting 30 percent of your total calories from protein. Be careful to mix the kinds of protein you eat so that you consume high-fat and high-purine proteins with low-fat and low-purine proteins. Choose from this list of proteins when deciding on a meal or snack.

High Purine: organ meats (pâté, liver, etc.), herring, mussels, sardines, anchovies

Moderate Purine: beef, bacon, dark meat chicken, duck, lamb, spareribs, dark meat turkey, veal, wild game, salmon, shellfish (lobster, shrimp, crab), oysters, scallops, octopus, squid, dark tuna, eggs, regular-fat cheeses

Low Purine: white meat chicken, turkey breast, lean pork, catfish, cod, flounder, perch, sole, trout, white tuna, swordfish, low-fat cheese, low-fat cottage cheese, skim milk, low-fat yogurt, egg whites

Carbohydrates

With regard to carbs, the real significant difference between balanced, fast, and slow oxidizers is not the types of carbs allowed, but the quantity. You should get 40 percent of your nutrients from carbs, but like everyone you should avoid simple carbs and foods that are rated high on the glycemic load index, which we get into in the next chapter. Refined sugars like those found in cookies, sweets, and soda, and processed grains like white bread or white rice should be shunned whenever possible, especially on a weight-loss regimen. You do best with a mix of fruits and vegetables from both the fast and slow oxidizers' carb lists.

Vegetables — Low Starch: asparagus, cauliflower, celery, mushrooms, spinach, broccoli, Brussels sprouts, cabbage, collard greens, cucumbers, garlic, kale, leafy greens, onions, peppers, scallions, sprouts, tomatoes, watercress

Vegetables — Moderate: Starch beets, eggplant, jicama, okra, yellow squash, and zucchini

Fruits: apples, berries, cherries, citrus fruits, peaches, pears, apricots, plums, tropical fruits

Grains: barley, brown rice, buckwheat, corn, couscous, kasha, millet, oat, quinoa, rice, rye, spelt

Legumes/Lentils (all fresh, nothing dried), tempeh, tofu, beans, peas

Fats

In order to best support your metabolism, you need to be getting roughly 30 percent of your calories from natural oils and fats. Don't eat excessive amounts of fat, but don't specifically restrict your fat intake. You can choose from fats on both the fast and slow oxidizers' lists of permissible fats.

Nuts/Seeds: (listed in order of protein content) walnuts, pumpkin seeds, peanuts, sunflower seeds, sesame seeds, almonds, cashews, Brazil nuts, filberts, pecans, chestnuts, pistachios, coconut, macadamias

Fats/Oils: butter, cream, almond oil, peanut oil, coconut oil, sesame oil, flaxseed oil, sunflower oil, walnut oil

Eat the foods that are ideal for you. Also remember these guidelines of what not to do.

1. Don't eat meals made up of just one macronutrient. Make sure you adhere to your ideal ratio of 40 percent carbs, 30 percent protein, and 30 percent fat.

2. Don't drink alcohol. It depletes glycogen storage in the liver, which causes an increase in blood sugar and fat storage. In addition, you will most likely experience a sugar crash, which leads to a heightened appetite for carbs and the nutrients you need to metabolize them. If you do have a drink, choose wisely and avoid sugary cocktails, beer, and wine. Opt instead for clear alcohols such as vodka or rum with calorie-free mixers, like club soda diet, light fruit juices or diet Snapple. And there's always straight or on the rocks as well.

3. Don't eat foods that are high on the glycemic load index. (Again, see the next chapter for a full understanding of glycemic load.) If you should happen to eat high-GLI foods, make sure you

accompany them with protein in order to show down the rate of oxidation and stabilize blood sugar and energy levels.

4. Don't drink too much caffeine. Caffeine is only effective as a fat burner or performance enhancer when taken in pill form and combined with aspirin. In the forms of coffee, tea, or soda, caffeine gives you short-term energy, but does that by signaling to your adrenal glands to dump their entire store out into your blood. When the caffeine wears off, your adrenal glands are so depleted they have to take a break, which means that you feel tired and weak.

5. Don't overcook your meat. Avoid overcooked animal products, since heat destroys essential amino acids and valuable enzymes.

Now that you have your list of foods that are ideal for your metabolic type, you will have more energy and feel better if you eat to support your metabolism. However, many of the foods on your list are high in calories. Your diet should incorporate these types of foods in accordance with your caloric allowance.

Metabolic Typing Test #2

Metabolic type tests will help determine the ratio of protein, carbohydrates and fats that are best for your weight loss effort. Using the results, it will be easier to understand how you should be eating to stay healthy and lose excess weight. You must understand why certain foods are ideal so that you can then make the best choices for your personal meal plan. The two ways to determine metabolic type are through a blood test or with a questionnaire.

1. I sleep best when:

(A) I eat 1-2 hours before going to sleep.

(B) I eat as much as 3-4 hours before going to sleep.

2. I sleep best if:

(A) My dinner is composed of mainly meat with some vegetables or other carbohydrates.

(B) My dinner is composed mainly of vegetables or other carbohydrates and a comparatively small serving of meat.

3. I wake up feeling well rested if

(A) I don't eat sweets, sugar or sugary snack in the evening.

(B) I eat sweets, sugar or sugary snack in the evening.

4. In the morning, I am

(A) Hungry and ready to eat breakfast.

(B) Not hungry and don't feel like eating.

5. I feel best during the day if I eat

(A) Small meals frequently, or three meals a day plus some snacks.

(B) Two to three meals a day and no snacks; I can last pretty long without eating.

6. I feel best when the temperature is

(A) Cool or cold; I don't like hot weather.

(B) Warm or hot; I don't like cold weather.

7. After vigorous exercise, I tend to crave:

(A) Foods or drinks with higher protein and/or fat content, such as a high-protein shake.

(B) Foods or drinks higher in carbohydrates (sweeter), such as Gatorade®, soda, or fruit juice.

8. At midday, I am

(A) Hungry and ready to eat lunch.

(B) Not noticeably hungry and have to be reminded to eat.

9. During the day, I feel hungry

(A) Often and need to eat several times a day.

(B) Rarely and have a weak appetite.

10. I describe myself as someone who

(A) Loves to eat; food is a central part of my life. Live to eat.

(B) Is not very concerned with food; I may forget to eat at times. Eat to live.

11. Instinctively, I prefer to eat:

(A) Dark meat, such as the chicken or turkey legs and thighs over the white meat breast.

(B) Light meat, such as the chicken or turkey breast over the dark meat leg and thigh.

12. In general, I prefer to:

(A) Salt my foods most of the time.

(B) Taste my foods and apply salt once in a while, but am not particularly attracted to salty foods.

13. If I skip a meal, I feel

(A) Irritable, jittery, weak, tired, or depressed.

(B) Okay; it doesn't really bother me.

14. If I attended a buffet and could eat whatever I wanted (all health rules aside), I would choose

(A) Steak, pork chops ribs, gravy, and a salad with creamy dressing.

(B) Chicken, turkey, fish, vegetables, and a dessert.

15. In order to last 4 hours between meals and maintain mental clarity and a sense of well-being, I prefer to eat:

(A) A meal predominantly meat-based, high in protein and fat (such as roast beef, pork, salmon…) with carbohydrate as a supplement to the meal.

(B) A meal predominantly carbohydrate base, such as a salad or vegetables with some bread, and a small amount of protein.

16. When I eat sugar or a sugary snack such as candy, jelly donuts or sweetened drinks,

(A) I feel a rush of energy, may get the jitters or may feel good for a short time, but then am likely to crash and feel fatigued.

(B) My energy levels are restored. I don't seem to be negatively affected, even though I know that too much is not good for me.

17. If dessert is served,

(A) I can take it or leave it; I would rather have cheese, chips, or popcorn.

(B) I definitely will indulge; I like to have something sweet after a meal.

18. My body shape is closest to:

(A) Mesomorphic or "V" shaped, like a typical wrestler, gymnast or weight lifter type; or Endomorphic or more naturally round shaped, but I am naturally quite strong and respond very well to anaerobic sports or strength training type exercises.

(B) Ectomorphic or long and lean like a rower or triathlete; or Endomorphic or more naturally round shaped, but I respond better to endurance athletics than to strength training or anaerobic sports.

Scoring – first by counting how many A and Bs you have marked down from the questions. Determine your metabolic type

- If your A score is 5 or more points higher than your B score (e.g., A = 11, B = 7), then you are a Protein Type.

- If your B score is 5 or more points higher than your A score (e.g., A = 7, B = 11), then you are a Carb Type.

- If your A and B scores are within 3 points of each other (e.g., A = 10, B = 8), then you are a Mixed Type.

Metabolic Type Test #3

Characteristic	Column 1	Column 2	Column 3
Aging	Look older than others my age	Look younger than others my age	
Aloofness	Cool, distant, aloof, loner, slow to make friends, hard to get to know	Warm, open, expressive, easily make friends, approachable	
Appetite	Weak, lacking, diminished	Strong, excessive, enhanced	Average appetite
Chest Pressure		Tend to get	
Climate	Love warm, hot weather	Do well in cold, poor in hot	Doesn't matter
Cold sores and/or fever blisters		Tend to get	
Coughing		Tend to cough most everyday	
Cracking Skin (any weather)		Tend to get	
Dandruff		Tend to get	
Desserts	Love sweets, need something sweet with meal to feel satisfied	Don't really care for sweet desserts, but like something fatty or salty (like cheese, chips or popcorn) for snacks after meals	Can take them or leave them
Digestion	Poor, weak, slow	Good, strong, rapid	Average digestion

Characteristic	Column 1	Column 2	Column 3
Eating before bed	Usually worsens sleep, especially if heavy food	Usually improves sleep	Doesn't matter, but heavy snacks are not the best
Eating Habits	Eat to live – unconcerned with food and eating	Live to eat-need to eat often to feel good, be at best	Average eating habits and need for food, meal times, etc…
Emotional Expression	Hard to express feelings, not naturally demonstrative	Easily express feeling	
Emotions	Beneath the surface, under control, non-emotional type, tend to hold feelings inside	Wear heart on sleeve, others always know how I feel	
Eye Moisture	Tend toward dry eyes	Tend toward moist or tearing eyes	
Facial Coloring	Tend toward pale, chalky	Tend toward ruddy, rosy, flushed	
Facial Complexion	Tend toward dull, unclear	Tend toward bright, clear	
Fatty food (if you like or dislike, not what you think is good for you).	Don't care for it.	Love it, crave it, would like it often.	Take it or leave it.
Fatty food reaction	Decreases energy and well-being	Increases well-being	Average reaction
Fingernails	Tend to be thick, hard, strong	Tend to be thin, soft, weak	

Characteristic	Column 1	Column 2	Column 3
4 Hours without eating	Doesn't bother	Makes me irritable, jittery, weak, famished or depressed	Feel normal hunger
Gooseflesh	Tend to form easily		
Gum Bleeding		Tend to get after Brushing	
Gum Color	Light Pale	Dark, pink, red	
Hunger Feelings	Rarely get, passes quickly, can easily go long periods without eating	Often hunger, need to eat regularly and often	When late for meals only, not between meals usually
Insect bite/sting	Weak reaction, disappears fast	Strong, lasting reaction	
Itching Eyes		Tend to get	
Itching Skin		Tend to get	Average reaction
Juice or Water Fasting	Can handle very well, feels good	Fasting makes me feel awful	React okay, can fast if necessary
Meal Portions	Prefer small	Prefer large, or if not large, need it often	Average
Orange Juice alone	Energizes, satisfies me	Can make me light-headed, hungry, jittery, shaky or nauseated	No ill effects
Potatoes	Not real fond of them	Could eat them almost every day, love them	Take them or leave them

Characteristic	Column 1	Column 2	Column 3
Red meat, like a steak or roast beef meal	Decreases energy and well-being	Increases well-being, energy	Average reaction
Saliva Amount	Tend toward dry mouth	Excessive saliva	
Saliva Texture	Tends to be thick, ropy	Tends to be thin, watery	
Salty Foods	Foods often taste too salty	Really love or crave salt on foods	Average like for it
Skin Healing	Cuts heal slowly	Cuts heal quickly	Average healing time
Skin Moisture	Tend toward dry skin	Tend toward oily/moist skin	Average skin moisture
Skipping Meals	Can skip with no ill effects	Must eat regularly (or often)	Can get by without eating but really feel best eating 3 meals per day
Snacking	Rarely or never want to snack	Want to eat between meals	
Sneezing (any time)		Tend to sneeze every day	
Sour foods (vinegar or pickles or lemons or sauerkraut or yogurt)	Don't care for, want, or crave	Really like	Sometimes like this flavor
Sweets	Can do fairly well on	Don't do well on, sweet foods can seem too sweet	No noticeable bad effect

Characteristic	Column 1	Column 2	Column 3
Vegetarian Meal	Is satisfying	Not satisfying, or bad result, become hungry soon after or feel unsatisfied	Okay, but not really satisfied
Wheezing		Tend to get	
If I eat MEAT for BREAKFAST like ham, bacon, sausage, steak or salmon	I get tired, sleepy, lethargic and/or very thirsty by midmorning	I feel great, energetic, have good stamina, and keeps me going without getting hungry before lunch.	It's okay, but not in large proportions
If I eat MEAT for LUNCH like hamburger, steak, roast beef or salmon	I get tired, sleepy, lethargic and/or lose my energy in the afternoon	I feel great, energetic, have good stamina, keeps me going without getting hungry before dinner	It's okay, but not in large proportions
If I feel low on energy	Fruit, pastry, or candy restores and gives me lasting energy; meat or fatty food makes me more tired.	Meat or fatty food restores my energy, fruit pastry or candy makes me worse…quick lift followed by a crash	Pretty much any food restores my energy
In a social setting I'm	Introverted, shy, quiet, non-talkative	Extroverted, social, expressive, easily make conversation	
TOTALS:			

CHAPTER NINE
PLANNING YOUR DAILY MEALS USING THE FACTS

By now you should have a pretty good idea about your Metabolic Type. I provided three different Metabolic Typing Tests above for you to use on different days so that you could ensure that you chose the right type. Why would I provide multiple tests? Your answers to the questions may actually differ from day to day, so multiple tests can ensure accuracy.

What Metabolic Type Are You?

After you've taken each of the tests above, you'll want to tally the number of A's, B's, and C's to determine which Metabolic Type you are. After you've figured your answers on each test, you'll want to choose which "type" you answered most often. For instance, if you answered Type A on two or more tests, that is more than likely the actual type that you are. Perhaps you chose Type B or Type C more often than the others. Depending upon your final "Metabolic Type," you'll want to begin creating your daily menus using foods from the lists that are also provided.

Having said that, let's begin creating!!!

Let's Review the Best Protein-Carbohydrate-Fat Ratios for You

For every Metabolic Type, there are foods that are better for the body chemistry that you should choose when preparing your menus. In other words, your body will work more efficiently, allowing you to burn more fat than if you eat the wrong foods and/or combinations of them.

To make planning your menus easier, I'm providing you with a few quick reference guides from which to choose each type of food, along with healthy serving sizes, too.

Identify What Foods will Work Ideally for You

Using the Metabolic Type that you determined was best for you, let's begin reviewing the foods best suited, as well as the appropriate serving size(s) that will produce the best results. Whether you are trying to lose, maintain, or gain weight, these foods will help you achieve your goals.

When using the charts below, find your Metabolic Type and then choose foods that appeal to your pallet.

Additionally, the sections that are shaded are considered to be the "best bet" food items for your Metabolic Type.

Protein Choices: Carbohydrate Types

Meats	Serving Size
Bacon (Pork)	1 Slice
Bacon (Beef)	1 Slice
Beef	1 Ounce
Buffalo	1 Ounce
Lamb	1 Ounce
Liver (Beef or Chicken)	1 Ounce
Pork (Lean)	1 Ounce
Rabbit	1 Ounce
Venison	1 Ounce

Poultry	Serving Size
Bacon (Turkey)	1 Slice
Chicken (Dark)	1 Ounce
Chicken (White)	1 Ounce
Duck	1 Ounce
Goose	1 Ounce
Cornish Hen	1 Ounce
Pheasant	1 Ounce
Quail	1 Ounce
Sausage (Chicken)	1 Ounce
Turkey (Dark Meat)	1 Ounce
Turkey (White Meat)	1 Ounce

Seafood	Serving Size
Abalone	1 Ounce
Anchovy	1 Ounce
Bass (Freshwater)	1 Ounce
Bass (Sea)	1 Ounce
Catfish	1 Ounce
Caviar	1 Ounce
Clams	1 Ounce

Seafood (continued)	Serving Size
Cod	1 Ounce
Crabmeat	1 Ounce
Crayfish	1 Ounce
Flounder	1 Ounce
Grouper	1 Ounce
Halibut	1 Ounce
Herring	1 Ounce
Lobster Meat	1 Ounce
Mackerel	1 Ounce
Mahi-mahi	1 Ounce
Mussels	1 Ounce
Octopus	1 Ounce
Perch (Freshwater)	1 Ounce
Rockfish	1 Ounce
Roughy	1 Ounce
Salmon	1 Ounce
Sardines	1 Ounce
Scallops	1 Ounce
Shark	1 Ounce
Shrimp	1 Ounce
Snapper	1 Ounce

Seafood (continued)	Serving Size
Squid	1 Ounce
Swordfish	1 Ounce
Trout	1 Ounce
Tuna (White)	1 Ounce
Whitefish	1 Ounce

Dairy and Eggs	Serving Size
Egg	1
Cottage Cheese (Raw)	¼ cup
Greek Yogurt	6 Ounces

Nuts & Seeds	Serving Size
Almonds	½ Ounce
Brazil Nuts	½ Ounce
Cashews	½ Ounce
Chestnuts	½ Ounce
Filberts	½ Ounce
Hickory Nuts	½ Ounce
Macadamia Nuts	½ Ounce
Peanuts *	½ Ounce

Nuts & Seeds (continued)	Serving Size
Pecans	½ Ounce
Pine Nuts	½ Ounce
Pistachios	½ Ounce
Pumpkin Seeds	½ Ounce
Sunflower Seeds	½ Ounce
Walnuts	½ Ounce
Nut Butter *	1 tbsp

*All nuts and seeds must be raw. *Peanuts are legumes but are listed with tree nuts for ease of presentation. *Varieties of nut butter include almond, cashew, macadamia nut and walnut.

Protein Choices: Protein Types

Meats	Serving Size
Bacon (Pork)	1 Slice
Bacon (Beef)	1 Slice
Beef	1 Ounce
Buffalo	1 Ounce
Lamb	1 Ounce
Liver (Beef or Chicken)	1 Ounce
Pork (any cut)	1 Ounce
Rabbit	1 Ounce
Venison	1 Ounce

Poultry	Serving Size
Bacon (Turkey)	1 Ounce
Chicken (Dark Meat)	1 Ounce
Chicken (White Meat)	1 Ounce
Cornish Hen	1 Ounce
Duck	1 Ounce
Goose	1 Ounce
Pheasant	1 Ounce
Quail	1 Ounce
Sausage (Chicken)	1 Ounce
Turkey (Dark Meat)	1 Ounce
Turkey (White Meat)	1 Ounce

Seafood	Serving Size
Abalone	1 Ounce
Anchovy	1 Ounce
Bass (Freshwater)	1 Ounce
Bass (Sea)	1 Ounce
Catfish	1 Ounce
Caviar	1 Ounce

Seafood (continued)	Serving Size
Clams	1 Ounce
Cod	1 Ounce
Crabmeat	1 Ounce
Crayfish	1 Ounce
Grouper	1 Ounce
Halibut	1 Ounce
Herring	1 Ounce
Lobster Meat	1 Ounce
Mackerel	1 Ounce
Mahi-mahi	1 Ounce
Mussels	1 Ounce
Octopus	1 Ounce
Perch (Ocean)	1 Ounce
Pompano	1 Ounce
Rockfish	1 Ounce
Roughy	1 Ounce
Salmon	1 Ounce
Sardines	1 Ounce
Scallops	1 Ounce
Shark	1 Ounce
Shrimp	1 Ounce

Seafood (continued)	Serving Size
Snapper	1 Ounce
Squid	1 Ounce
Swordfish	1 Ounce
Trout	1 Ounce
Tuna (Dark)	1 Ounce
Whitefish	1 Ounce

Dairy & Eggs	Serving Size
Egg	1
Cottage Cheese (Raw)	¼ Cup
Greek Yogurt	6 Ounces

Nuts & Seeds	Serving Size
Almonds	½ Ounce
Brazil Nuts	½ Ounce
Cashews	½ Ounce
Chestnuts	½ Ounce
Filberts	½ Ounce
Hickory Nuts	½ Ounce
Macadamia Nuts	½ Ounce

Nuts & Seeds (continued)	Serving Size
Peanuts *	½ Ounce
Pecans	½ Ounce
Pine Nuts	½ Ounce
Pistachios	½ Ounce
Pumpkin Seeds	½ Ounce
Sunflower Seeds	½ Ounce
Walnuts	½ Ounce
Nut Butter *	1 tbsp

*All nuts and seeds must be raw. *Peanuts are legumes but are listed with tree nuts for ease of presentation. * Varieties of nut butter include almond, cashew, macadamia nut, and walnut.

Carbohydrate Choices: Carbohydrate Types

Bread	Serving Size
SWG Bread	1 Slice
SWG Roll	½
SWG English Muffin	1
SWG Wrap (Small)	1
Rice Bread	1 Slice
Spelt Bread	1 Slice
Rice Crackers	10
Rye Crackers	2

Grains	Serving Size
Brown or Wild Rice	½ Cup
Amaranth	½ Cup
Barley	½ Cup
Buckwheat	½ Cup
Corn	½ Cup
Kamut	½ Cup
Millet	½ Cup
Oatmeal	1 Cup
Quinoa	½ Cup
Rye	½ Cup
Spelt	¼ Cup
SWG Cereal	½ Cup
Raw Granola	½ Cup

Fruits	Serving Size
Apple (Medium)	1
Apricots (Small)	4
Banana (Medium)	½ Cup
Blackberries	1 Cup
Blueberries	1 Cup

Fruits (continued)	Serving Size
Boysenberries	1 Cup
Cantaloupe	1 Cup
Casaba Melon	1 Cup
Cherries	17
Cranberries	1 Cup
Currants	1 Cup
Date	1
Elderberries	¾ Cup
Figs (Large)	2
Gooseberries	1 Cup
Grapefruit (Small)	1
Grapes	17 – 20
Guava	1 Cup
Honeydew Melon	1 Cup
Kiwifruit (Medium)	2
Kumquat	6
Lemons	Free
Limes	Free
Loganberries	1 Cup
Mango	½
Nectarines (Small)	2

Fruits (continued)	Serving Size
Orange (Large)	1
Papaya (Large)	½
Peach (Medium)	1
Pear (Medium)	1
Persimmons	2
Pineapple	1 Cup
Plums (Small)	2
Pomegranate (Small)	1
Prunes (Small)	4
Raisins	¼ Cup
Raspberries	1 Cup
Rhubarb	2 Cups
Strawberries	1 Cup
Tangerines (Small)	2
Tomato (Large)	1
Watermelon	1 Cup

Legumes	Serving Size
Adzuki Beans	½ Cup
Black Beans	½ Cup
Black-Eyed Peas	½ Cup
Fava Beans	½ Cup
Garbanzo Beans	½ Cup
Great Northern Beans	½ Cup
Green Beans	½ Cup
Green Peas	½ Cup
Lentils	½ Cup
Lima Beans	½ Cup
Mung Beans	½ Cup
Navy Beans	½ Cup
Pink Beans	½ Cup
Pinto Beans	½ Cup
Red Beans	½ Cup
White Beans	½ Cup

High-Starch Vegetables	Serving Size
Beets	1 Cup
Carrots	1 Cup
Jerusalem Artichoke	½ Cup
Parsnips	½ Cup
Potato (White)	½ Cup
Potato (Sweet)	½ Cup
Water Chestnuts	¼ Cup

Low-Starch Vegetables	Serving Size
Artichoke	1
Asparagus	1 Cup
Bamboo Shoots	½ Cup
Bok Choy	1 Cup
Broccoli	1 Cup
Brussels Sprouts	1 Cup
Cabbage	1 Cup
Cauliflower	1 Cup
Celery	1 Cup
Cucumber	1 Cup
Daikon	1 Cup

Low-Starch Vegetables (continued)	Serving Size
Eggplant	1 Cup
Fennel	1 Cup
Garlic	Free
Ginger root	Free
Jicama	1 Cup
Kale	1 Cup
Lettuce	Free
Mushrooms	1 Cup
Okra	1 Cup
Olives	5
Onion (Medium)	1
Pepper (Bell)	1 Cup
Pepper (Hot)	1 Cup
Pumpkin	½ Cup
Radishes	½ Cup
Rutabaga	½ Cup
Salad Greens	1 Cup
Spinach	1 Cup
Squash (Winter)	½ Cup
Turnip	½ Cup
Zucchini	1 Cup

Dairy	Serving Size
Milk (Raw)	½ Cup
Plain Yogurt	6 Ounces

Notes: Serving sizes of grains and legumes are measured cooked; those of fruits and vegetables are measured raw. SWG – sprouted whole grains (e.g. Ezekiel 4:9 products); Free – Use as needed for seasoning.

Carbohydrate Choices: Protein Types

Bread	Serving Size
SWG Bread	1 Slice
SWG Roll	½
SWG English Muffin	1
SWG Wrap (Small)	1
Rice Bread	1 Slice
Spelt Bread	1 Slice
Rice Crackers	10
Rye Crackers	2

Grains	Serving Size
Brown or Wild Rice	½ Cup
Amaranth	½ Cup
Barley	½ Cup
Buckwheat	½ Cup
Corn	½ Cup
Kamut	½ Cup
Millet	½ Cup
Oatmeal	1 Cup
Quinoa	½ Cup
Rye	½ Cup
Spelt	½ Cup
SWG Cereal	½ Cup
Raw Granola	½ Cup

Fruits	Serving Size
Apple (Medium)	1
Apricots (Small)	4
Avocado	2 Ounce
Banana (Medium)	½
Blackberries	1 Cup
Blueberries	1 Cup

Fruits (continued)	Serving Size
Boysenberries	1 Cup
Cantaloupe	1 Cup
Casaba Melon	1 Cup
Cherries	17
Cranberries	1 Cup
Currants	1 Cup
Date	1
Elderberries	¾ Cup
Figs (Large)	2
Gooseberries	1 Cup
Grapefruit (Small)	1
Grapes	17 – 20
Guava	1 Cup
Honeydew Melon	1 Cup
Kiwifruit (Medium)	2
Kumquat	6
Lemons	Free
Limes	Free
Loganberries	1 Cup
Mango	½ Cup

Fruits (continued)	Serving Size
Nectarines (Small)	2
Orange (Large)	1
Papaya (Large)	½
Peach (Medium)	1
Pear (Medium)	1
Persimmons	2
Pineapple	1 Cup
Plums (Small)	2
Pomegranate (Small)	1
Prunes (Small)	4
Raisins	¼ Cup
Raspberries	1 Cup
Rhubarb	2 Cups
Strawberries	1 Cup
Tangerines (Small)	2
Tomato (Large)	1
Watermelon	1 Cup

Legumes	Serving Size
Adzuki Beans	½ Cup
Black Beans	½ Cup
Black-Eyed Peas	½ Cup
Fava Beans	½ Cup
Garbanzo Beans	½ Cup
Great Northern Beans	½ Cup
Green Beans	½ Cup
Green Peas	½ Cup
Lentils	½ Cup
Lima Beans	½ Cup
Mung Beans	½ Cup
Navy Beans	½ Cup
Pink Beans	½ Cup
Pinto Beans	½ Cup
Red Beans	½ Cup
White Beans	½ Cup

High-Starch Vegetables	Serving Size
Beets	1 Cup
Carrots	1 Cup
Jerusalem Artichoke	½ Cup
Parsnips	½ Cup
Potato (White)	½ Cup
Potato (Sweet)	½ Cup
Water Chestnuts	¼ Cup

Low-Starch Vegetables	Serving Size
Artichoke	1
Asparagus	1 Cup
Bamboo Shoots	½ Cup
Bok Choy	1 Cup
Broccoli	1 Cup
Brussels Sprouts	1 Cup
Cabbage	1 Cup
Cauliflower	1 Cup
Celery	1 Cup
Cucumber	1 Cup
Daikon	1 Cup
Eggplant	1 Cup

Low-Starch Vegetables (continued)	Serving Size
Fennel	1 Cup
Garlic	Free
Gingerroot	Free
Jicama	1 Cup
Kale	1 Cup
Lettuce	1 Cup
Mushrooms	1 Cup
Okra	1 Cup
Olives	5
Onions (Medium)	1
Pepper (Bell)	1 Cup
Pepper (Hot)	Free
Pumpkin	½ Cup
Radishes	½ Cup
Rutabaga	½ Cup
Salad Greens	1 Cup
Spinach	1 Cup
Squash (Winter)	½ Cup
Turnip	½ Cup
Zucchini	1 Cup

Dairy	Serving Size
Whole Milk (Raw)	½ Cup
Plain Yogurt	6 Ounce

Notes: Serving sizes of grains and legumes are measured and cooked; those of fruits and vegetables are measured raw. SWG – sprouted whole grain (e.g., Ezekiel 4:9 products). Free – Use as needed for seasoning.

Mixed Metabolic Type

Remember, if you find your "type" a part of this group, you are able to use both the charts for Protein Type choices as well as the charts for Carbohydrate Type choices when choosing the foods that are best suited for you.

Fat Choices: All Metabolic Types

Fat	Serving Size
Olive Oil	1 tsp
Fish Oil	1 tsp
Cod Liver Oil	1 tsp
Flax Seed Oil	1 tsp
Raw Butter	1 tsp
Avocado	1 ounce
Coconut Oil	Free
Raw Cheese	1 ounce

Note: The fat content of foods that are considered fatty such as eggs, meats, oily fish and nuts have been accounted for in the allotted serving sizes and calories for each Metabolic Type, so no separate fat servings need to be calculated for these foods.

Planning Your Menu:

Now that you've determined the "Metabolic Type" that your body adheres to, you'll want to begin planning your meals. Part of planning your meals will include a few basics. For instance, you'll want to know the ideal food ratios for your metabolic type; you'll need to know the allowable servings (recommended) for your body type in order for you to lose weight. This is important and something that you won't want to eliminate from your meal planning routine in order to insure the successes that you hope to achieve. By closely following the program outlined, you'll be able to meet and/or achieve your weight loss goals.

Ideal Food Ratios for Each Metabolic Type

When attempting to lose weight, it helps to know the food ratios that will help you achieve your weight loss goals. Here are a few quick reference charts to assist you along the way. When using these charts, be sure to choose the correct Metabolic Type for you. Each chart reflects the proportion of foods that you should consume within each category of food types.

Ideal Food Ratios:

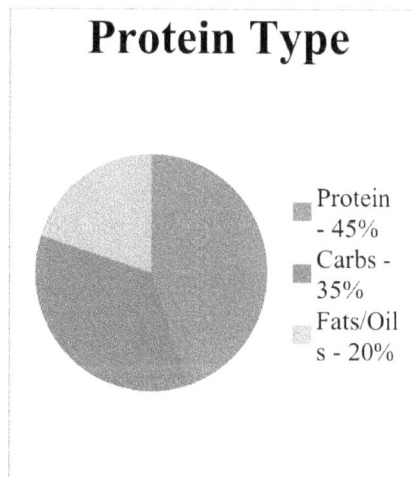

Protein Type

Protein - 45%
Carbs - 35%
Fats/Oils - 20%

Carbohydrate Type

- Carbs - 70%
- Protein - 20%
- Fats/Oils - 10%

Mixed Type

- Protein - 40%
- Carbs - 50%
- Fats/Oils - 10%

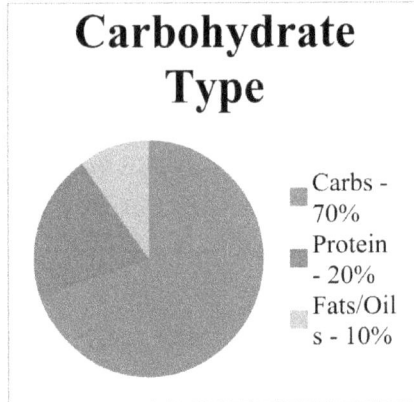

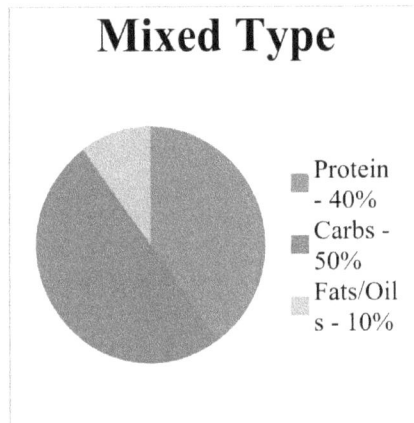

Allowable Servings Guide:

Another chart that you may find valuable in your weight loss quest is the Allowable Servings Guide. This chart will help you to determine, based on the number of calories per day that your body needs, the number of servings per meal based on your Metabolic Type. Hopefully you'll find this guide easy to use so that you can get started right away planning your meals.

1400 Calories Per Day			
Type	Mixed	Carbohydrate	Protein
Meal			
Breakfast	2 Protein/2 Carb.	1 Protein/2 Carb.	3 Protein/1 Carb.
Snack	2 Protein/2 Carb	1 Protein/2 Carb.	2 Protein/1 Carb.
Lunch	3 Protein/1 Carb/1 Fat	3 Protein/2 Carb/1 Fat	3 Protein/1 Carb/2 Fat
Snack	2 Protein/1 Carb.	2 Protein/2 Carb.	2 Protein/ 1 Carb.
Dinner	3 Protein/2 Carb/2 Fat	3 Protein/2 Carb/1 Fat	4 Protein/1 Carb/2 Fat

1600 Calories Per Day			
Type	Mixed	Carbohydrate	Protein
Meal			
Breakfast	2 Protein/2 Carb.	1 Protein/2 Carb.	3 Protein/1 Carb.
Snack	2 Protein/2 Carb	1 Protein/2 Carb.	2 Protein/1 Carb.
Lunch	4 Protein/1 Carb/1 Fat	4 Protein/2 Carb/1 Fat	4 Protein/1 Carb/2 Fat
Snack	2 Protein/1 Carb.	2 Protein/2 Carb.	2 Protein/ 1 Carb.
Dinner	4 Protein/2 Carb/2 Fat	4 Protein/2 Carb/2 Fat	4 Protein/2 Carb/1 Fat

1800 Calories Per Day			
Type	Mixed	Carbohydrate	Protein
Meal			
Breakfast	2 Protein/2 Carb.	1 Protein/2 Carb.	3 Protein/1 Carb.
Snack	2 Protein/2 Carb	2 Protein/2 Carb.	3 Protein/1 Carb.
Lunch	4 Protein/2 Carb/1 Fat	4 Protein/2 Carb/1 Fat	4 Protein/1 Carb/2 Fat
Snack	2 Protein/1 Carb.	2 Protein/3 Carb.	2 Protein/ 1 Carb.
Dinner	5 Protein/2 Carb/2 Fat	4 Protein/2 Carb/1 Fat	5 Protein/1 Carb/2 Fat

2000 Calories Per Day			
Type	Mixed	Carbohydrate	Protein
Meal			
Breakfast	3 Protein/2 Carb.	2 Protein/3 Carb.	3 Protein/1 Carb.
Snack	2 Protein/2 Carb	2 Protein/2 Carb.	3 Protein/1 Carb.
Lunch	4 Protein/2 Carb/1 Fat	4 Protein/2 Carb/1 Fat	5 Protein/1 Carb/2 Fat
Snack	2 Protein/1 Carb.	2 Protein/3 Carb.	3 Protein/ 1 Carb.
Dinner	5 Protein/2 Carb/2 Fat	4 Protein/2 Carb/1 Fat	5 Protein/1 Carb/2 Fat

2200 Calories Per Day			
Type	Mixed	Carbohydrate	Protein
Meal			
Breakfast	3 Protein/2 Carb.	2 Protein/3 Carb.	4 Protein/1 Carb.
Snack	3 Protein/2 Carb	2 Protein/3 Carb.	3 Protein/1 Carb.
Lunch	4 Protein/2 Carb/1 Fat	4 Protein/3 Carb/1 Fat	5 Protein/1 Carb/2 Fat
Snack	2 Protein/2 Carb.	2 Protein/3 Carb.	4 Protein/ 1 Carb.
Dinner	5 Protein/2 Carb/2 Fat	4 Protein/2 Carb/1 Fat	5 Protein/1 Carb/2 Fat

2400 Calories Per Day			
Type	Mixed	Carbohydrate	Protein
Meal			
Breakfast	3 Protein/2 Carb.	2 Protein/3 Carb.	4 Protein/2 Carb.
Snack	3 Protein/2 Carb	2 Protein/3 Carb.	3 Protein/1 Carb.
Lunch	4 Protein/3 Carb/2 Fat	4 Protein/3 Carb/2 Fat	5 Protein/1 Carb/2 Fat
Snack	3 Protein/2 Carb.	2 Protein/3 Carb.	4 Protein/ 1 Carb.
Dinner	5 Protein/2 Carb/2 Fat	4 Protein/3 Carb/1 Fat	6 Protein/1 Carb/2 Fat

Note: In order to make the most of these charts/guides, you'll want to refer to the appropriate foods in each category for your Metabolic Type.

Glycemic Index Guide

If you watch any television at all, you've seen the commercials for many of the world's leading food substitution and weight loss programs touting the importance of the Glycemic Index. Simply put, the Glycemic Index measures how fast and how much a food raises blood glucose levels. Foods with higher index values raise blood sugar more rapidly than foods with lower Glycemic Index values do. Why is this significant in weight loss?

The body breaks down most carbohydrates contained in foods we eat and converts them to a type of sugar called glucose. Glucose is the main source of fuel for our cells. After eating, the time it takes for the body to convert carbohydrates and release glucose into the bloodstream varies, depending on the type of carbohydrate and the food that contains it. Some carbohydrate-containing foods cause the blood glucose level to rise rapidly; others have a more gradual effect.

When attempting to lose weight, you want your blood glucose levels to remain constant or at least fluctuate very little so that your body is not triggered to store fat. By eating combinations of foods that will level off your glucose level, your body doesn't behave in ways that we'd rather it not.

Glycemic Index Chart

	Index	Sugar	Dairy	Fruit	Grain	Vegetables
High	>100	Maltose; Beer; Alcohol		Date		Parsnip
High	90 – 99	Glucose; Sports Drinks			Instant Rice; Puffed Rice	
High	80 – 89	Jelly Beans			Rice Chex, White Rice, Pretzels, Rice Krispies, Corn flakes, Rice Cakes	Potato (White, Baked); Potato (White, Instant Mashed)
High	70 – 79	Life Savers; Jams; Jellies		Watermelon	Wheat Cereal; Graham Crackers; Cheerios; Bagels; Whole Wheat Bread; White Bread; Millet	Pumpkin; Rutabaga
Medium	60 – 69	Honey		Melon (all types); Pineapple; Raisin; Banana (ripe); Apricot; Mango	Cornmeal; Rye Crisp Bread; Shredded Wheat; Brown Rice; Brown Rice Pasta	Beet
Medium	50 – 59			Kiwifruit	Corn; Popcorn; Oatmeal;	Potato (sweet); Yam; Carrot;

	Index	Sugar	Dairy	Fruit	Buckwheat Grain	Green Peas Vegetables
Low	40 - 49	Lactose		Grape; Orange	Wheat Bran; Bulgur Wheat; Whole Wheat Pasta	Beans (Pinto or Baked)
Low	30 - 39		Yogurt; Whole Milk; Butter	Apple; Pear; Strawberry	Rye	Tomato Soup; Beans (Navy, Lima, Black, or Garbanzo); Peas (Black- eyed or dried split)
Low	<30	Fructose		Peach; Grapefruit; Plum; Cherry; Tomato	Barley; Rice Bran	Beans (Kidney or lentil); peas (dried); Eggplant; Summer Squash; Cauliflower; Peanut; Green Vegetables

Note: On the Glycemic Index Scale, high-GI foods are rapid insulin inducers and should be avoided; low GI foods are slow insulin inducers and your best choices for weight loss.

Vegetables with a GI of 15 are ideal carbohydrates and include: artichoke, asparagus, broccoli, celery, cucumber, green beans, lettuce, green bell pepper, spinach and zucchini.

Source: Adapted from Wolcott and Fahey 2000, 272 – 274.

Sample Menu: Protein Type

You've done it. You've made it through one of the most important books that you'll ever read and/or need in your quest to achieve your weight loss goals. By closely studying the information provided, and implementing the information provided in the Charts and Guides, you can now customize your menu(s) to be used during mealtimes.

But, before you get started on planning your own menus, allow me to share with you a few sample menus so that you'll see just how easy it is to create a menu using the recommended portions, choosing foods from the appropriate food charts.

Let's begin with a Protein Type Meal Menu:

Sample Menu: Protein Type

Meal	Food	Serving Size		
		Protein	Carb	Fat
Breakfast	2 eggs (poached or scrambled)	2		
	1/3 cup dry oatmeal (in hot cereal with cinnamon		1	
Snack	1 oz cashews	2		
	1 medium pear		1	
Lunch	5-6 oz beef, ground (in a burger or chili)	6		
	½ cup cooked kidney beans (in chili)		1	
	Small green salad or ½ cup raw vegetables		½	
	Apple cider vinegar + 1 tsp olive oil			1
	1 tsp (or 2 softgels) fish oil or cod liver oil			1
Snack	2 tbsp walnut or almond butter	2		
	8 oz celery sticks and carrot sticks		1	

Meal	Food	Serving Size		
		Protein	Carb	Fat
Dinner	5-6 oz chicken, dark meat (baked or grilled)	6		
	½ cup spinach (sautéed)		½	
	¼ cup cooked couscous		½	
	Small green salad		½	
	Apple cider vinegar + 1 tsp olive oil			1
	1 tsp (or 2 softgels) fish oil or cod liver oil			1

Note: Fish Oils contain the long chain of Omega-3 fatty acids like DHA and EPA. They provide the body with the most anti-inflammatory and heart-healthy ingredients available in a supplement formula.

Sample Menu: Carbohydrate Type

Meal	Food	Serving Size		
		Protein	Carb	Fat
Breakfast	2 slices turkey bacon	2		
	½ cup cooked millet or quinoa (in hot cereal)		1	
	½ large grapefruit		1	
Snack	½ oz almonds (raw)	1		
	½ large grapefruit		1	
Lunch	4 oz chicken (grilled)	4		
	¼ cup cooked kamut		½	
	½ cup cooked lentils		1	
	½ cup cooked broccoli (steamed or sauteed)		½	
	Small green salad		½	
	Apple cider vinegar + 1 tsp olive oil			1
Snack	1 tbsp walnut butter	1		
	4 oz celery sticks		½	
	20 grapes		2	
Dinner	4 oz shrimp or scallops (grilled or baked)	4		
	½ cup green vegetables (stir-fried)		½	
	½ cup cooked brown rice		1	
	Small green salad or ½ cup raw vegetables		½	

150 ▪ Randa Lee Roberts

Meal	Food	Serving Size		
		Protein	Carb	Fat
	Apple cider vinegar			
	1 tsp (or 2 softgels) fish oil or cod liver oil			1

Note: Fish Oils contain the long chain of Omega-3 fatty acids like DHA and EPA. They provide the body with the most anti-inflammatory and heart-healthy ingredients available in a supplement formula.

Sample Menu: Mixed Type

Meal	Food	Serving Size		
		Protein	Carb	Fat
Breakfast	2 eggs (in an omelet)	2		
	1 cup chopped raw spinach, peppers, and onions (in an omelet)		1	
	1 slice SWG bread		1	
	1 medium pear		1	
Snack	1 oz almonds or walnuts	2		
	1 medium apple		1	
	1 cup cucumber slices		1	
Lunch	4 oz turkey, ground white and dark meat (in a burger)	4		
	8 oz carrot sticks		1	
	½ cup cooked brown rice		1	
	Small green salad		½	
	1 tsp (or 2 softgels) fish oil or cod liver oil			1
	Apple cider vinegar			
Snack	1 – 2 tsp peanut or almond butter	2		
	2 slices rye crisp bread		1	
	8 oz celery sticks		1	
Dinner	5 oz halibut steak (broiled)	5		

Meal	Food	Serving Size		
	½ cup green beans (sautéed with garlic)		½	
		Protein	Carb	Fat
	4 oz sweet potato (baked)		1	
	Small green salad or ½ cup raw vegetables		½	
	Apple cider vinegar + 1 tsp olive oil			1
	1 tsp (or 2 softgels) fish oil or cod liver oil			1

Note: SWG = sprouted whole grain (e.g., Ezekiel 4:9 products). Fish Oils contain the long chain of Omega-3 fatty acids like DHA and EPA. They provide the body with the most anti-inflammatory and heart-healthy ingredients available in a supplement formula.

Let's Get Started:

Now that you've had an opportunity to review the sample menus for each Metabolic Type, what are you waiting for? It's time to start planning your meals. Remember, these are three separate menus for three different metabolic types, so you'll see some repetition. Do not think for one minute that you need to replicate these menus or include the same items for each meal. Variety is the spice of life, and I've provided you plenty of food choices to choose from.

CHAPTER TEN
CREATING YOUR MEAL PLANS

Now that you've reviewed all of the facts that are going to assist you in creating a healthy meal plan for your Metabolic Type, let's get started. In this section I've provided you with blank meal plan charts so that you can simply fill in the details for your food selections choosing foods that you enjoy. These charts can be duplicated for your use.

Blank Meal Plan Chart:

Meal	Food	Serving Size		
		Protein	Carb	Fat
Breakfast				
Snack				
Lunch				

Meal	Food	Serving Size		
		Protein	Carb	Fat
Snack				
Dinner				

Notes: Use this space to include any recipes or notes that you need to keep on track.

CHAPTER ELEVEN
FOOD FACTS TO CONSIDER WHEN PLANNING YOUR MEALS

Beginning a lifestyle modification can be somewhat scary – especially the first couple of steps. Luckily for you, you're way past the first few steps. So far, you've discovered the secrets about certain foods that should be included and excluded from your daily dietary consumption; you've learned about farming practices that truly do make the difference; you've discovered that not all sweeteners are created equal; and about your specific Metabolic Type, which will allow you to put into place a plan that will be effective.

Having said all of that, it's time to start planning your meals. Perhaps you'd prefer that the first couple were carefully planned for you. That would be great, except that every individual reading this book will more than likely have different desires in terms of the foods chosen to make their individualized plan(s) successful. Since I cannot establish individualized diets for everyone, allow me to share a few recipes that have been tried, tested, and are true for your use if you find them appealing to your pallet.

Before jumping into menus, however, let me share with you a few food facts that I want to ensure you remember BEFORE you begin cooking.

Food Facts:

In the beginning of this manual, I shared with you LOTS of information about healthy vs. not so healthy food choices that individuals make on a daily (if not hourly) basis. This will simply be a short review for quick reference.

Organic IS Best!!!

As you begin your healthy lifestyle makeover and modification, you'll want to consider making the change to organic vs. the other guys. You will notice a significant difference not just in the flavor of the organic foods, but your body will notice a significant difference too. For starters, choose organic, free-range poultry, meat, eggs, and MILK. Most organic varieties can be found in your local supermarket; however, if you're unsuccessful shopping there, visit a local health food store. A few stores that I know carry organic selections are: Publix, Kroger, Whole Foods, Market Fresh, and Costco. If you have none of these stores within or near your community, you can order products online at www.grasslandmeats.com.

If you are unable to obtain organic foods when shopping, your next best bet would be to select foods that are free-range, antibiotic, and hormone-free. You'll be able to read these details on the labels, and this will apply to poultry, meats and eggs.

Next on your shopping list will be organic produce. If you'll recall, I provided you a list of produce that will have more pesticide residues than others. If you're living on a budget, like so many of us do these days, begin replacing produce that contains the most residue first. A quick list of those foods includes: vegetables such as spinach, celery, potatoes, hot and bell peppers; and fruits such as nectarines, red raspberries, strawberries, apples, peaches, cherries, imported grapes, and pears.

The Facts on Fat(s):

I know the word "fat" sounds like it will defeat the purpose of dieting. Fortunately, it is a necessary evil in the world of weight loss. The body MUST have fat in order to burn it. The detail is in the type of fat that your body needs in order to do its job. So without further ado, let's tackle some of the facts.

Plan an afternoon to purge your cupboards. You're going to be reading labels on foods and ingredients that contain hydrogenated or partially hydrogenated oils. You'll be surprised at the number of items you're going to be tossing – in fact, you may think to yourself, "That's a lot of food wasted!" Well, that depends on your ultimate goal. Prepackaged foods, including chips, crackers, cookies, cereal bars, cereals, microwave popcorn, and anything labeled low-fat and fat-free will need to find their way into the trash can or be donated to a local food bank (as it will provide food for those who otherwise may not have any). It's that important.

You'll need to rewire your mind to recognize what snacks should be vs. what we're preprogrammed to think they are. Snacks are no longer chips, crackers, cookies, or popcorn. Those types of snacks should be replaced with healthier alternatives and should be "mini-meals" of the healthier foods that you'll be eating regularly. These choices may include hard-boiled eggs (I eat them every day), a few pieces of chicken or turkey with vegetables, chopped vegetables such as carrots, celery, cucumbers, or other wonderful choices from the food charts provided, fruits, and nuts or nut butters. Fresh food is always more beneficial for you, so choose wisely.

You'll have to use some form of fat for cooking, so choose quality fats instead of the cheaper varieties that will be offered at your grocer. Choose coconut oil and raw organic butter. You cannot go wrong with these selections. Organic extra virgin olive oil is preferred and can always be used for sautéing, or used raw, as in salads.

Avoid margarine and other processed butter spreads, as these will undoubtedly contain hydrogenated vegetable oil.

Each and every day you'll want to consume at least two or three servings of Omega-3 fats from fish oil, seeds (flaxseeds), avocados, or nuts (raw, organic, and unsalted), most notably walnuts. Remember, roasted nuts should be avoided, as the roasting process results in the fats and oils becoming rancid. Rancid oils increase free-radical damage in the body (which can accelerate aging).

Organic nut butters are an excellent choice that can be added to almost any meal. More often than not you can find peanut, almond, cashew, and macadamia nut butters in stores. When selecting nut butters at your grocer you'll want to READ THE LABEL. They should contain only nut(s) and salt. Peanut butters are often made of roasted peanuts, and we know that cannot be good for us.

When cooking with fat(s), always add them to a cold pan and increase the heat gradually. This will decrease the likelihood of scorching the fats.

Milk! It Does a Body Good – Or Does It? And Other Dairy Products

This one will be a tough one, but one that you should carefully consider when choosing dairy products. If you are a regular, daily dairy product consumer, try to secure raw (unpasteurized) certified organic products. You may have to find a local producer in order to do this as regulations make it difficult to obtain. However, if you cannot obtain raw, then choose the next best thing – certified organic. These products will still be homogenized or pasteurized (perhaps both), but they'll lack antibiotics, hormones, and pesticide residues.

Although you may feel as though you cannot eliminate dairy from your diet, just know that most of the calcium obtained from these products isn't absorbed by the body anyway, meaning that your body can go without these products to avoid the unhealthy elements. You can obtain calcium from other healthy sources such as green leafy vegetables, sardines (bones included), broccoli, and salmon.

Don't Be Fooled by Advertising – Avoid Soy Products

During your cupboard eviction event, discard any product containing soy protein isolate, soy protein concentrate, texturized vegetable protein, or soy (soybean oil). Products containing these ingredients will include: mayonnaise, pre-packaged energy bars, crackers, vegetable burgers, and other vegetarian products.

If you, like so many others, have been consuming "soy-based or containing" products for an extended period of time, you may want to visit your doctor and have your thyroid checked. It may be functioning improperly as a result of soy exposure. Hypothyroidism may be the result, and by eliminating soy products from your diet, you may see positive changes in your condition.

"Step Away from that Loaf" – Grains & Breads

Grains can be the culprits of so many things – from allergies and bloating, to sharp increases in glucose levels, to weight gain. In order to choose the healthiest grains and breads, choose those containing only sprouted whole grain products. Two excellent choices are Ezekiel 4:9 Food for Life (found in the freezer section), and Manna bread. Try using original sesame and cinnamon raisin loaves, rolls, English muffins, and tortillas. These are all excellent choices and can be used to make breadcrumbs for recipes needing them. Another alternative would be breads and bread-type products made from rice or spelt.

Breakfast and lunch do NOT require bread so try not to feel the need to include them. Focus on your Metabolic Type and choose foods such as eggs, fruits, and nut butters for breakfast. Choose salads or vegetables with poultry, fish, or other meat options for lunch.

If you experience unexplained gastrointestinal distress (gas & bloating) it may be a sign that you are gluten-intolerant. Simply eliminate all gluten grains from your diet for 4 to 6 weeks to see if the condition improves.

A Sprinkle a Day – Salt

Many people crave it, while others despise it! Salt – an unnecessary evil. If you are one of the many people who cannot live without that salty flavor on your foods and sprinkle it like a thunderstorm is upon you, you may want to reconsider. Avoid ALL refined white table salt and avoid ALL high-sodium packaged and canned foods. (In fact, if you read labels, you'll be shocked to discover how much sodium is contained within.)

In lieu of refined table salt you'll want to choose unprocessed, unrefined sea salt for all of your cooking and flavoring needs. Although there are plenty on the market, the two best choices are: Celtic Sea Salt or Redmond's Real Salt. As mentioned above, there are many variations out there; unfortunately, they may contain mercury or other toxic heavy metals.

Read the labels – if it says unprocessed and unrefined, it is a better choice.

Note: In order to avoid adding too much salt, salt AFTER the food is prepared and always taste it first.

H2O a.k.a. Water

You would think that as important as water is to the body that ALL of it would be safe to drink. You've probably heard the statement when referring to consuming the water in Mexico, "Don't Drink the Water!" But have you ever considered the water in your neck of the woods? Knowing how much water and what kind is important NO MATTER where you are.

There are a few simple rules of thumb when it comes to clean, safe drinking water. First and foremost, if you are on city water or water that is supplied via a water processing plant, know that there will ALWAYS be byproducts associated with prescription drugs present. Metals, additives, toxins, and other elements will be included, which is why I have a filtration system at my home. There are filters available for your entire house or for your water faucets, bath water, AND ice makers. Choose carefully. If you are concerned about the quality of the water being provided, contact your city/county and request a report. They must test and release the results annually.

If you're on well water, there are also elements present. Have your well tested regularly so that you can determine the byproducts and metals that are present. You, too, may want to consider a filtration system.

Once you've determine the safety and quality of the water that you're consuming, you'll want to remember to drink enough water daily to allow your body to perform optimally. Everyone should drink ½ of their body weight (pounds) in ounces of water each day. For instance: if you weigh 160 pounds – divide that in half to reach 80 and you'll want to consume 80 ounces of water each day.

For each caffeinated beverage consumed, you should drink 8 ounces of water.

If you exercise during the day, you should drink 8 ounces of water to help replenish your balance.

If you're feeling hungry (or think you're hungry), drink 8 ounces of water to help you determine if you're actually hungry or dehydrated.

To reduce the risk of overeating at mealtimes, drink 8 ounces of water 15 minutes before each meal.

Plastic water bottles should ALWAYS be kept out of the sun and away from heat to avoid leaching of toxins from the plastic into the water.

All Sweeteners are NOT Created Equally!

One of my biggest pet peeves these days is everything is sweetened to death! Read the labels of everything that you or your loved ones will consume!!! The saying "buyer beware" should only pertain to real estate purchases. You'd be surprised at the dangers (and toxins) included in many consumable products.

When reading labels, the sugar content will be listed beneath the carbohydrate listing such as:

Nutrition Facts	
Serving Size	2 Tbsp (37g)
Calories	70
Fat Calories	0
Total Fat	1g
Sodium	290mg
Total Carbohydrates	16g
Sugars	14g

It is also a wise practice to read the ingredients contained within the product – the order (sequence) in which the ingredients are listed will provide insight into the relative quantity of the ingredient. An example would be as listed on a popular salad dressing: Soybean Oil, Water, Egg Yolk, Sugar, Salt, Cultured Nonfat Buttermilk, Natural Flavors (Soy), Spices, etc., compared to another popular barbeque sauce: High Fructose Corn Syrup, Distilled Vinegar, Tomato Pesto, Water, Modified Food Starch, Molasses Corn Syrup, Garlic, Sugar, Tamarind, Natural Flavor.

Avoid foods containing artificial sweeteners, sugars, or sugar derivatives such as Equal, Sweet & Low, Splenda (aspartame, saccharin, Sucrolose, and all sugar alcohols.)

Many beverages these days include sweeteners. Read labels and choose drinks that avoid any form of extra sugar.

For your sweetening needs, use Stevia.

Bartender, May I Have Another… The Dangers of Alcohol

While alcohol consumption is enjoyed by millions of people around the world, it isn't a preferable beverage when attempting to lose weight and modify your lifestyle. If you CANNOT go without, it is suggested that you drink no more than one glass per week.

If you drink alcohol, organic red wine is best. The rich flavor will encourage you to drink it slowly. Red wine contains fewer calories and carbohydrates than other types of alcohol.

If wine isn't your thing and you feel the need to consume alcoholic beverages, vodka is the second choice. Served on the rocks; fruit juice will add only empty sugar calories. When choosing brands, Chopin is considered the best, as it is made from potatoes, not wheat!

Once you've established your ideal weight (or reached your weight goals), you can be more lenient with alcohol consumption, but minimizing it will help to maintain a healthy weight.

PART THREE

Tips & Tools to Make Your Transition Easier

CHAPTER TWELVE
HEALTHY RECIPES TO MAKE PLANNING MENUS EASIER

Healthy recipes are sometimes hard to come by, so I'm going to provide you with a sampling of healthy recipes for various items that you'll want to keep close at hand when preparing meals for your friends, family, and loved ones.

Beverage(s):

Flavored Tea(s)

This beverage is a healthy alternative to sugar-laden drinks that you may crave.

5 – 6   bags of decaffeinated tea (any brand) preferably herbal teas (e.g., peach, mint, chamomile, raspberry, or other fruit variety)

3 quarts boiling water

Stevia powder (or liquid) to taste. (Honey can be used instead)

Directions: Pour water over tea bags in a large pot. Add Stevia while tea is hot. (Adjust amount according to desired taste).

Let cool, remove tea bags, transfer to pitcher, refrigerate.

Garnish with a slice of fresh fruit and/or berries.

Acai Berry and Pomegranate Smoothie
Serves: 4
(recipe by Jillian Michaels, Master Your Metabolism)

1 (3-1/2 ounce)	packet frozen acai berry puree, partially thawed
1 cup	pomegranate juice
1 cup	low-fat plain kefir
2 scoops	whey protein powder
1 tablespoon	agave syrup (stevia powder or honey)
2 cups	ice cubes (about 8 cubes)

Directions: In blender, place the acai berry puree, pomegranate juice, kefir, whey protein powder, agave syrup (Stevia powder or honey), and ice. Cover and blend until smooth.

Divide among four glasses and serve.

Enjoy!

Banana-Almond Smoothie

Serves: 2

1 cup	sliced banana (use 1 large banana)
1 cup	almond milk
1 tablespoon	almond butter
1 tablespoon	ground flaxseed
1 tsp	vanilla extract
2 cups	ice cubes (about 8 cubes)

Directions: Place banana, almond milk & butter, flaxseed, and vanilla in blender. Blend until very well combined, approximately 45 to 60 seconds. Add ice cubes and blend until smooth.

Pour into (2) glasses and serve.

Dressings, Marinades, Seasonings and Sauces

Make it Your Own Salad Dressing

Makes: ¾ Cup

1 tsp	dijon mustard, smooth or grainy
2 Tbsp + 1 tsp	wine vinegar
½ cup	extra virgin olive oil
1 Tbsp	flaxseed oil

Directions: Whisk mustard into vinegar. Add olive oil in a thin stream, whisking constantly until oil is emulsified. Whisk in flaxseed oil (Omega-3's).

Serve Immediately.

Variation: Mix 1 tsp finely chopped fresh herbs (e.g. parsley, basil, tarragon, thyme, rosemary, oregano) into the recipe after the mix is emulsified. For a spicier rendition, add 1/8 tsp of fresh horseradish.

Lemon Pepper Dressing

Makes: ¾ cup
(recipe by Joseph Mercola, Dr. Mercola's Total Health Program)

2 Tbsp	fresh-squeezed lemon juice
1 Tbsp	wine vinegar
¼ tsp	Celtic Sea Salt
½ tsp	cracked black peppercorns
1 dash	Stevia powder (honey)
1 clove	minced (fresh) garlic
½ cup	extra virgin olive oil
1 Tbsp	flaxseed oil

Directions: Whisk all ingredients in bowl until emulsified.
Serve Immediately.

Good for Everything Marinade

This recipe is so versatile that it can be used on fresh vegetables, fish, poultry, and beef. An excellent addition to London Broil.

Preparation Time: 15 Minutes
Marinating Time: Overnight
Makes: Enough for 20 pounds of food

1	red onion (sliced)
1	head of garlic (cloves, minced)
4 tsp	Celtic Sea Salt
4 tsp	ground white pepper
4 tsp	fresh ground pepper
4 tsp	paprika
3 tsp	basil (dried) – although I prefer fresh
4 tsp	Worcestershire sauce
1 cup	fresh-squeezed lemon juice
1-1/4 cups	red wine vinegar
4 cups	olive oil (32 ounces)

Directions: Mix all ingredients until well blended. Pour over food to be marinated. Marinate overnight.

Caribbean Jerk Rub

Dry rubs are low-calorie, low-carbohydrate seasonings that are simple and very flavorful. This recipe is great on grilled Caribbean Chicken. **(Recipe by Joseph Mercola, Dr. Mercola's Total Health Program)**

6 Tbsp	Minced garlic (or garlic powder – NOT SALT)
6 Tbsp	Minced onion
6 Tbsp	dried minced onion (or onion powder)
2 Tbsp	allspice
1 Tbsp	dried, ground chipotle (or ground red chili pepper – fresh is BEST)
2 Tbsp	Hungarian paprika
1 Packet	Sweet Leaf Stevia Powder (or honey)

2 Tbsp	dried thyme
2 Tbsp	ground cinnamon
2 tsp	ground nutmeg
1-1/2 tsp	ground habañera pepper
Zest	2 lemons

Mix together the ingredients above. This can be stored in a covered container, if refrigerated, up to 1 month.

Béarnaise Sauce

When preparing this lovely sauce, never expose to anything more than medium heat. In keeping the heat low, the enzymes in the egg yolks are preserved.

Delicious served on or beside meats and grilled fish. (Recipe by Sally Fallon, Nourishing Traditions)

Makes: 1-1/4 Cup

2 Tbsp	finely chopped shallots (or green onions)
1 Tbsp	finely chopped fresh tarragon (or 1 tsp dried tarragon)
2 Tbsp	white wine vinegar
2 Tbsp	dry white wine (or vermouth)
5	egg yolks (room temperature)
4 oz (1 stick)	unsalted butter, cut into pieces

Fresh lemon juice to taste

Pinch of Celtic Sea Salt

Pinch of freshly ground black pepper

Directions: In small saucepan, combine the shallots, tarragon, vinegar, and wine. Bring to boil and reduce, leaving 1 Tbsp of liquid. Strain into a small bowl and set aside.

In another bowl, whisk egg yolks and set aside.

Set the bowl with the reduced liquid over a pan of hot water over low heat (double-boiler works well). Piece by piece, add about half of the butter to the liquid, whisking constantly until melted. Add the egg yolks slowly, drop by drop or in a thin stream, whisking constantly. Add the remaining butter and whisk until well amalgamated. Sauce should be warm and slightly thickened. Remove from heat and whisk in lemon juice, salt and pepper.

Set the bowl over hot water to keep sauce warm, whisking occasionally, until served.

Fruit Vinaigrette

Makes: ¾ Cup or 6 (2) Tbsp Servings

This sweet-and-savory vinaigrette is so versatile. Use with fresh fruit, makes a great dressing for salad greens, and excellent with chopped vegetables, grilled fish, or poultry.

1 cup	chopped fruit, i.e., pineapple, mango, blueberries, raspberries, orange, tangerine, or grapefruit.
1 Tbsp	extra-virgin olive oil
1 tsp	balsamic vinegar

Directions: In blender, place the fruit, olive oil, vinegar and up to 2 teaspoons of water. Blend until smooth and pourable, adding more water (1 teaspoon) at a time as necessary to thin the mixture. Use at once or store in a tightly covered container in the refrigerator for up to 3 days.

Homemade Vegetable Broth

Makes: 2 Quarts

Vegetable broths found on the market today are less than satisfying in terms of flavor. Creating your own base will certainly add to the overall flavor of your finished product.

1	large yellow or red onion (peeled)
1	garlic clove (peeled and halved)
2	large carrots cut into 2-inch pieces
2	celery stalks, cut into 2-inch pieces
8 oz	button or cremini mushrooms, coarsely chopped
2	small turnips or 1 fennel bulb (coarsely chopped)
6	fresh parsley sprigs

| 4 | fresh thyme sprigs |
| 1 | fresh or dried bay leaf |

Directions: In stockpot, place the onion, garlic, carrots, celery, mushrooms, and turnips. Tie the parsley, thyme, and bay leaf together (for seasoning only) with kitchen string and add to the pot. Add 2 quarts of cold water, or enough to cover the vegetables. Partially cover the pot and bring the water to a boil over medium-high heat. Reduce the heat and skim any foam from the surface. Simmer gently, partially covered, for 1 hour.

Strain the broth through a fine-mesh strainer. Do not press on the vegetables or the broth will become cloudy. Let cool (room temperature). Broth can be stored in a tightly sealed container for up to 3 days in the refrigerator or in the freezer for up to 6 months.

Marinara Sauce:

Makes: 4 Cups (Serves 8)

Although you may be tempted to purchase prepared marinara sauce while shopping, a quick review of the ingredients may surprise you, as it isn't uncommon for them to be loaded with sugar or high-fructose corn syrup. Making your own is not only cheaper, but allows you to control every ingredient that goes into it.

1 Tbsp	virgin olive oil
1 cup	finely chopped red onion
2	garlic cloves (finely chopped)
1	fresh or dried bay leaf
¼ cup	tomato paste (choose organic)
1 (28 oz)	can low-sodium crushed tomatoes (or crush your own fresh tomatoes)
1 Tbsp	chopped fresh parsley, or 1 tsp dried
1 Tbsp	chopped fresh basil, or 1 tsp dried
1 tsp	balsamic vinegar
1/4 tsp	Celtic Sea Salt
¼ tsp	Ground black pepper

Directions: In large skillet or heavy-bottomed pan, heat the olive oil over medium heat (do not overheat). Add the onion, garlic, and bay leaf and cook, stirring, until softened and beginning to brown – approx. 6 – 8 minutes.

Move the onion and garlic to one side of the pan and add the tomato paste to the cleared spot. Cook for about 2 minutes. Stir the onion and garlic into the paste and continue to cook, stirring occasionally, until the paste is darker in color – approx. 2 – 3 minutes.

Stir in the crushed tomatoes, parsley, oregano, Balsamic vinegar, and salt & pepper. Increase the heat to medium and bring to a boil. Reduce the heat and simmer for 15 minutes. Remove and discard the bay leaf.

If a smooth sauce is desired, transfer the sauce to the work bowl of a food processor or blender and process until the desired consistency is obtained.

Serve warm. For longer storage, let the sauce cool and transfer to a tightly sealed container. Can be stored in the refrigerator for up to 4 days or in the freezer for 6 months.

Ketchup:
Makes: 2 Cups (32 – 1 Tbsp servings)

Another of the seriously over processed staples found at the grocer is ketchup. It isn't uncommon for it to be described at red-colored corn syrup. This recipe is one that is sure to delight your pallet and contains wholesome ingredients.

3 Tbsp	olive oil (plus a little extra for the pan)
2 Pounds	ripe plum tomatoes cut lengthwise in half
1 tsp	whole allspice
1 tsp	whole cloves
1 (3 inch)	cinnamon stick
1 cup	chopped red onion
2	garlic cloves (chopped)
1 Tbsp	tomato paste (again, choose organic)
2 Tbsp	maple syrup
1 Tbsp	cider vinegar
¼ tsp	Celtic Sea Salt

Set a rack 6 inches below the broiler and heat the broiler to high. Brush a rimmed baking sheet with olive oil.

Place the tomatoes cut side down on the baking sheet. Brush the tomatoes with 2 Tbsp of the olive oil. Broil until they are softened and brown in spots, approx. 8 – 10 minutes (watch closely). Remove from the oven and set the pan aside.

Lay a double layer of unbleached cheesecloth on the work surface. Place the allspice, cloves, and cinnamon stick in the center. Bundle them in the cheesecloth and tie it tightly with kitchen string. Set aside. Alternatively, you can toss all the spices directly into the pot, but be sure to fish them all out before you puree the ketchup.

In a Dutch oven or other large, heavy-bottomed saucepan, heat the remaining 1 Tbsp of olive oil over medium-low heat. Add the onion and garlic and cook, stirring occasionally until softened, approx. 8 minutes. Stir in the tomato paste and cook, continuing to stir occasionally, for 2 minutes. Add the reserved tomatoes and their juice, the maple syrup, vinegar, salt and spice bundle. Cover and cook for 5 minutes. Remove the cover and simmer for 30 minutes.

Remove and discard the spice bundle (or fish out the spices mentioned above). Transfer the mixture to the work bowl of a food processor or blender and puree until smooth. Clean out the Dutch oven and return the puree to it. Simmer until thickened and reduced, approx. 50 minutes to 1 hour, stirring occasionally.

Let cool before serving. Store the ketchup in a tightly sealed container in the refrigerator for 1 week or freeze for up to 6 months. Once you've discovered the exceptional flavor, you may choose to purchase multiple storage containers so that you can always have extra in the freezer.

Soy-Free Mayonnaise

If you'll recall, soy products aren't considered good for you. In fact, I devoted a great deal of page space talking about soy and soy products, just in case you want to review the information provided. I'll bet you didn't know that commercially produced mayonnaise is a soy-based product. Yes, every last jar at the grocery store begins with soy this or that. So, I've developed a recipe for mayonnaise that tastes better than national brands, takes less than 10 minutes to create, AND is soy-free.

2 Tbsp + 2 tsp   vinegar OR lemon juice

2	egg yolks (or pasteurized powdered egg yolks)
½ tsp	Celtic Sea Salt
1 tsp	Mustard
1 tsp	Stevia powder or honey
2 cups	light extra virgin olive oil (heavy olive oil is too overpowering)

Directions: In a food processor (speeds up the production time) or a mixing bowl, mix the vinegar (or lemon juice) with the salt, mustard, and Stevia (or honey). Add the egg yolks (or egg yolk mixture according to preparation directions.) Pulse several times until everything is well-blended.

Add about 1 tsp of the oil at a time while running the processor. Add the oil very slowly – this is important when making mayonnaise, or the mixture won't emulsify and you will end up with oily (too much liquid) instead of a creamy, smooth mixture. Take your time. If the mixture becomes too thick, add ½ teaspoon of water at a time until you reach the desired consistency.

This homemade recipe does not contain preservatives like store brands, so only make what you'll use within a seven-day period. Because it only takes 10 minutes to whip up, you can always make more when needed.

Variations: If desired, you can add a few fresh herbs or garlic as your palate will enjoy. Additionally, you can use as much or little of the lemon juice or vinegar as well to make it suit your individual taste(s). Finally, using spicy brown mustard gives it an extra kick when you want it.

Vegetable Dishes:

Summer Salad

Serves: 6

This salad is best served after it's been allowed to sit a few hours – it allows the flavors to blend.

¾ cup	lemon pepper dressing
1 bunch	celery, finely chopped
2	cucumbers (medium), peeled, quartered lengthwise, and finely chopped
2 bunches	green onions, finely chopped
2	green peppers, seeded and finely chopped
1 bunch	radishes, finely chopped
3	tomatoes (medium – large)
1 Tbsp	chopped fresh parsley or chives

Directions: Place dressing in a large bowl. Add celery, cucumbers, green onions, peppers, and radishes. Toss well with dressing and cover. Refrigerate several hours.

Just before serving, thinly slice the tomatoes, and cut slices in half. Arrange slices around the outer edge of six plates and mound the salad mixture in the center of each. Sprinkle with chopped parsley.

Wilted Spinach

Serves: 6

2 bunches	fresh spinach
1 Tbsp	butter (unsalted)
1	clove garlic, minced
1 Tbsp	pine nuts
1 Tbsp	sun-dried tomato flakes (optional)

Directions: Cut stems off spinach and wash well in water (even if prewashed) so that the leaves are moist. Place in a large pot, cover, and heat over medium (do NOT add water to the pot; the remaining water on the leaves from washing is all you'll need to steam the spinach).

When spinach begins to simmer, reduce heat to low. Cook several minutes until the leaves are wilted.

In a saucepan, melt the butter; add garlic, pine nuts and tomato flakes.

Using a slotted spoon, transfer the spinach to a serving bowl. Pour the mixture over the spinach to mix slightly and serve.

Tomatillo and Tomato Salsa
Makes: 2-1/2 Cups

½ pound	tomatillos (about 6), papery husks removed; rinsed and diced
½ pound	ripened, firm red tomatoes, diced
¼ cup	finely chopped red onion
1	small garlic clove, finely chopped
1	red or green fresh chili, such as jalapeño, serrano, or mirasol, seeded & minced
1/3 cup	fresh cilantro leaves, chopped
1 to 2 Tbsp	fresh lime juice
¼ tsp	Celtic Sea Salt
¼ tsp	ground black pepper

Directions: In medium bowl, combine the tomatillos, tomatoes, onion, garlic, and chili. Let stand at room temperature for 1 hour.

Stir in cilantro, lime juice, salt, and pepper.

This salsa can be stored in a tightly sealed container in the refrigerator for up to 4 days.

Coconut-Ginger Yellow Rice
Serves: 4

1 tsp	virgin coconut oil
1	shallot, chopped
1 tsp	turmeric

¼ tsp	Celtic Sea Salt
¼ tsp	ground black pepper
¾ cup	coconut milk
1 cup	long grain brown rice
4	lime wedges, for garnish

Thin quarter-size slice of fresh ginger.

Directions: In a medium saucepan, heat the oil over low heat. Add the shallot, turmeric, and salt and pepper. Cook, stirring occasionally, until the shallot begins to soften, approx. 1 – 2 minutes.

Stir in the coconut milk, ginger, and 1-1/4 cups water. Increase the heat to medium and bring to a boil. Stir in the rice and return to a boil. Reduce the heat, cover, and simmer gently until the rice is tender and the liquid is absorbed, approx. 45 – 50 minutes. Remove and discard the ginger and fluff with a fork just before serving. Garnish with lime wedges, if desired.

Serve.

Russet Potato Salad with Arugula and Lemon
Serves: 10

This is an excellent dish if you're entertaining – a perfect addition to summer picnics and family barbeques.

2 oz	arugula leaves, stems trimmed, leaves coarsely chopped (about 2 cups)
3 pounds	Russet potatoes, scrubbed and cut into ¾ inch pieces
1	large head of garlic, cloves separated and chopped
¾ tsp	Celtic Sea Salt
2 Tbsp	champagne vinegar
1 tsp	dijon mustard
1/3 cup	extra virgin olive oil
1 cup	chopped celery
3 Tbsp	chopped fresh chives or green scallions

Grated zest and juice of 1 lemon

Directions: Place the arugula in a large mixing bowl.

In a large saucepan, place the potatoes, garlic, and ¼ tsp of the salt; add cold water to cover. Bring to a boil. Reduce the heat and simmer, partially covered, until the potatoes are just tender, about 5 minutes. Drain well and transfer to the bowl with the arugula.

Meanwhile, pour the lemon juice into a glass measuring cup. Add enough vinegar to make ¼ cup. Pour into a small mixing bowl. Add the mustard, grated lemon zest, remaining ½ teaspoon of salt, and ¼ teaspoon of pepper. Whisk to combine. Whisking constantly, pour in the olive oil in a steady stream.

Pour the vinaigrette over the potatoes and toss gently. Set aside to cool for 30 to 60 minutes, and then refrigerate until cold.

Stir in the celery and chives. Taste for seasoning and add more lemon juice or pepper if desired.

Serve.

Spinach and Red Onion Quiche
Serves: 6

1	frozen whole-wheat pie crust, set at room temperature for 20 minutes
1 Tbsp	olive oil
½	medium red onion, thinly sliced
¼ tsp	Celtic Sea Salt
¼ tsp	ground black pepper
1	garlic clove, finely chopped
4 oz	Shiitake mushrooms, stems trimmed and discarded, caps thinly sliced
1 pound	fresh spinach, trimmed and coarsely chopped
3	large eggs
¾ cup	almond Milk
½ cup	grated Parmesan cheese

Pinch of freshly grated nutmeg

Preheat oven to 350 Degrees Fahrenheit.

Directions: Use a fork and prick the pie crust in several places to prevent bubbles. Bake until lightly browned, about 20 minutes. Remove from the oven and set aside.

Meanwhile, in a large skillet, heat the olive oil over medium-low heat. Add the onion and 1/8 teaspoon each of the salt and pepper. Cook, stirring occasionally, until softened, about 4 minutes. Add the garlic and cook until fragrant and lightly browned, about 30 seconds. Add the mushrooms and cook until softened, about 4 minutes. Add the spinach to the skillet and cook until wilted, approx. 1 – 2 minutes.

Transfer the spinach mixture to a colander. Press firmly with the back of a spoon to squeeze out as much liquid as possible. Transfer the spinach mixture to the crust and spread to cover. Place the crust pan on a rimmed baking sheet, if desired, to make it easier to transfer the quiche to the oven.

In a medium bowl, whisk together the eggs, almond milk, Parmesan, nutmeg, and remaining 1/8 teaspoons of both the salt and pepper. Pour the egg mixture over the spinach. Bake until the quiche is just set when the pan is gently nudged, 40 – 45 minutes. Let stand for 15 minutes before serving.

Serve.

Baked Ratatouille with Parmesan
Serves: 6

2 Tbsp	olive oil
1	medium eggplant (about ¾ pound) cut into ½ inch cubes
½ tsp	Celtic Sea Salt
1	medium red onion, diced
1 Tbsp	finely chopped garlic
¼ tsp	crushed red pepper flakes
1 Tbsp	tomato paste (choose organic)
2	red bell peppers cut into ½ inch cubes
1 (28 ounce)	can diced tomatoes, drained (choose organic) or use fresh
1	medium zucchini (about 6 ounces), cut into ¼ inch thick half-moons
1	medium summer squash (about 6 ounces), cut into ¼ inch thick half-moons
2 (15 ounce)	cans no-sodium chickpeas, rinsed and drained

1 Tbsp	chopped fresh thyme leaves or 1 tsp dried
1 Tbsp	chopped fresh marjoram leaves or 1 tsp dried
¼ tsp	ground black pepper
2 Tbsp	grated Parmesan cheese

Preheat oven to 450 degrees Fahrenheit. Have a 3-quart baking dish ready.

Directions: In a skillet over medium-high heat, heat 1 tablespoon of the olive oil until hot but not smoking. Add the eggplant and a pinch of the salt. Cook, stirring occasionally, until lightly browned, about 8 minutes. Spread the eggplant in the bottom of the baking dish.

Wipe the skillet clean and heat the remaining 1 tablespoon of olive oil over medium-low heat. Add the onion, garlic, and red pepper flakes and cook, stirring occasionally, until softened, about 4 minutes. Stir in the tomato paste and cook for about 1 minute more. Add the peppers and cook until softened, about 8 minutes.

Stir in the drained tomatoes, the zucchini, summer squash, chickpeas, thyme, marjoram, remaining salt, and pepper. Bring to a boil, cover, and simmer for 5 minutes.

Spoon the mixture evenly over the eggplant. Sprinkle the cheese evenly over the top. Bake until bubbling and lightly browned on top, about 30 minutes. Let stand for 10 minutes before serving.

Serve.

Black Bean Chili
Serves 6

2 cups	dried black beans
2 Tbsp	olive oil
2	medium onions, finely chopped
2	green bell peppers, cored, seeded, and finely chopped
6	garlic cloves, finely chopped
1 Tbsp	chili pepper
1 Tbsp	ground cumin
1 Tbsp	dried oregano
½ tsp	ground cinnamon

¼ tsp	ground black pepper
1 (28 ounces)	can diced tomatoes with their juice (choose organic)
1 tsp	grated orange zest
1 cup	fresh orange juice
1 Tbsp	honey (organic)
1 to 3 tsp	chopped chipotle chilies in adobo (optional)
½ cup	medium-grind bulgur
½ tsp	Celtic Sea Salt

Garnish:

½ cup	nonfat plain Greek yogurt
3 Tbsp	minced scallions (white and green parts)
3 Tbsp	minced fresh cilantro
8	lime wedges

Directions: Place the beans in a colander, removing any debris; rinse and drain. Place them in a Dutch oven or other large, heavy pot; add water to cover by 2 inches. Bring to a boil. Reduce the heat to low and simmer, partially covered, until almost tender, about 1 hour. Drain and set aside.

Heat the oil in the same large pot over medium-high heat until hot but not smoking. Add the onions and bell peppers and cook, stirring occasionally, until just starting to brown, 8 to 10 minutes. Stir in the garlic and cook until fragrant, about 30 seconds. Stir in the chili powder, cumin, oregano, cinnamon, and black pepper. Then stir in the tomatoes, orange zest and juice, honey, chipotle, and 3 cups water. Add the reserved beans. Return to a simmer and cook, partially covered, checking occasionally and adding more water as needed, until the beans are just tender to the bite, about 1-1/2 hours. Stir in the bulgur 15 minutes before removing the chili from the heat. Taste and add up to ½ teaspoon salt for flavor.

Divide the chili into eight bowls and top each serving with the yogurt, scallions, cilantro, and a lime wedge, if desired, or pass the toppings separately at the table.

Serve.

Homemade Sprouted Grain Ezekiel Bread:

Ingredients:
- 3½ cups of untreated/raw whole grains (try the following combination: ½ cup barley flour, ¼ cup finely ground broad bean (fava bean) flour, ¼ cup millet flour, 1 cup durum/spelt wheat flour, ½ cup finely ground lentil flour)
- 1 tablespoon vinegar
- 1½ teaspoons salt
- 2¼ teaspoons, or one ¼ ounce package active dry yeast

Instructions:
To make sprouted flours:
1. Place grains into a large bowl and cover with warm water by about two inches and then add vinegar. Stir together to combine.
2. Let the grains soak in the bowl for 18 to 24 hours, depending on the kind (see the chart below).
3. Drain the grains and rinse them well. Then place them in a shallow bowl/dish/container that has a wide opening in which air can circulate. You can add 1–2 tablespoons of water for moisture but the grains shouldn't be soaking anymore. Leave the grains out on the countertop in a room-temperature space.
4. Allow the grains to sit and sprout over 2–3 days (depending on the kind). Every 12 hours while they're soaking, rinse them well. Leave them to sprout until you see tiny, cream-colored sprout emerging at the end of the grains.
5. Once sprouted, rinse and dry grains. Transfer the grains to the oven or a dehydrator lined with nonstick sheets. Dehydrate the grains for 12 to 18 hours or until first. You can either freeze the grains to use later at this point, or grind them into flour/dough to use right away. To grind them to flour in order to bake into bread, follow directions below for making bread.

To make homemade bread:
1. Add about half of the grains to a food processor/grinder and sprinkle half the salt over. Process until the mixture comes together into a ball. Place it in an airtight covered container. If you want your bread to have a fermented sourdough taste, leave the container at room temperature for 1 to 2 days. If not, leave it out for no more than about 12 hours.

2. Add the yeast and knead the dough. Do this on a clean counter by sprinkling the dry yeast over the dough and kneading for no less than 20 minutes.

3. Allow the yeast to get active by transferring the dough to a bowl and forming it into a ball. Cover the bowl with a plastic bag and let it sit for about 1 ½ hours so the yeast and grains can interact, and the dough rill rise.

4. Preheat your oven to 350F (177C). Grease a bead pan and press in your dough. Bake for about 60 minutes (or if you have a thermometer, until the internal temperature of the bread measured reaches about 180 to 190F).

Storing the bread:

Because your bread will have no preservatives in it and sprouted flour is prone to growing mold over time, it's recommended to freeze your bread within 2–3 days of making it. You can also try making sprouted bread (or muffins, cookies, etc.) in bulk and freezing them for later.

Meat Entrees:

Grilled Caribbean Chicken

Serves: 5

(Recipe by Joseph Mercola, Dr. Mercola's Total Health Program)

Preparation Time: 10 Minutes

2	broiler-fryer chicken halves (certified organic)
1 Tbsp	coconut oil (or butter)
6 Tbsp	Caribbean Jerk Rub (previous recipe)

Preheat grill to medium.

Rub broiler-fryer halves lightly with oil and then with Caribbean Jerk Rub. Cook chicken, turning every 15 – 20 minutes until tender, approx. 1 to 1-1/2 hours.

Chicken Margarita

Serves: 4

1 tsp	ground cumin
1 Tbsp	chili powder
10	cloves garlic, finely chopped
3 Tbsp	olive oil, divided
3-1/2 lb	chicken pieces
½ cup	tequila, white or gold
½ cup	water

Juice of 3 limes
Fresh cilantro leaves (for garnish)

Directions: In a large bowl, combine cumin, chili powder, lime juice, garlic, and 1 teaspoon olive oil. Marinate chicken pieces in this marinade for 20 minutes.

In a heavy skillet, heat remaining olive oil. Brown chicken pieces on all sides. Add marinade, tequila, and water. Cook for approximately 10 minutes. Transfer chicken pieces to a platter. Reduce sauce over high heat until it thickens to a good coating consistency, pour over chicken, and serve garnished with cilantro.

Cornish Game Hens with Grapes

Serves: 4

(recipe by Sally Fallon, Nourishing Traditions)

Preheat oven to 375 degrees Fahrenheit.

2	Cornish game hens split lengthwise
2 Tbsp	olive oil
2 Tbsp	butter, melted
½ cup	dry white wine (or vermouth)
2 cups	chicken stock

| 2 cups | red (or green) seedless grapes |
| 2 Tbsp | arrowroot mixed with 2 tablespoons water. |

Celtic Sea Salt and freshly ground pepper to taste.

Note: Arrowroot is a fine white powder that resembles cornstarch. Because it thickens when heated in liquid, it is an excellent ingredient to use for thickening sauces.

Directions: Place game hens, skin side up, in a roasting pan. Brush with a mixture of butter and oil, and season with salt and pepper. Bake for about 1-1/2 hours. Remove to a heated platter, and keep warm in the oven. Pour wine into the roasting pan and bring mixture to a boil, scraping up any accumulated juices in the pan. Add chicken stock, bring to a rapid boil, skim, and let the sauce reduce for about 10 minutes. Add the grapes, and simmer about 5 minutes more. Add arrowroot mixture by the spoonful until the desired thickness is obtained. Transfer game hens to individual plates, and pour sauce over to serve.

Serve and Enjoy!

Roasted Turkey Breast with Cranberry-Orange Sauce
Serves: 8

1	boneless, skinless turkey breast (about 2-1/2 pounds)
2 tsp	chopped parsley
2 tsp	chopped fresh rosemary, plus sprigs for garnish
2 tsp	chopped fresh sage, plus sprigs for garnish
1 tsp	chopped thyme leaves
½ tsp	Celtic Sea Salt
¼ tsp	fresh ground pepper
1 Tbsp	olive oil
½ cup	fresh orange juice (from 1 to 2 oranges)
½ cup	fresh or frozen cranberries
2 tsp	honey

Up to ½ cup low-sodium chicken broth (or broth made from scratch).

Position oven rack to center of the oven. Preheat oven to 350 degrees Fahrenheit.

Directions: Place the turkey breast on a work surface skin side down. Holding a sharp knife parallel to the work surface, start at the middle of the breast and cut a deep incision into the thickest part of the meat, cutting toward the outer edge of the breast; be very careful not to cut all the way through. Open this flap like a book. Repeat the process on the other side. Open this flat out to the other side. Cover the turkey with a sheet of wax paper. Using the flat side of a meat mallet, pound the breast gently to flatten it evenly.

In a small bowl, combine the parsley, rosemary, sage and thyme. Sprinkle the herbs over the cut surface of the roast. Starting at a short end, roll the breast into a thick cylinder. Tie crosswise in three or four places with kitchen string. Season the outside of the roast with the salt and pepper.

In a Dutch oven or flameproof casserole dish slightly larger than the turkey breast, heat the olive oil over medium-high heat. Add the breast and cook, turning occasionally, until browned on all sides, about 10 minutes. Cover tightly and bake until an instant-read thermometer inserted in the center of the breast reads 160 degrees to 165 degrees Fahrenheit, about 30 minutes. Transfer the turkey breast to a carving board and loosely tent with aluminum foil to keep warm.

Pour the cooking juices out of the pot into a 1-cup glass measure. Let stand for a few minutes, and then skim off the fat that rises to the surface using a spoon or paper towels. Add enough chicken broth to the cooking juices to make ½ cup. Return the liquid to the pot and add the orange juice, cranberries, and honey. Bring to a boil over high heat. Boil until the cranberries have popped and the sauce is slightly thickened and has reduced to about 2/3 cup, about 5 minutes. Stir in any juices from the turkey.

Thinly slice the turkey and divide among eight plates. Pour the sauce over each plate and serve.

Pork Medallions with Pomegranate Sauce:

Serves: 4

Pomegranate is the greatest for disrupting the damaging effects of bad LDL cholesterol. That means that it will assist to keeping your arteries clear and your heart healthy. Having said this, let me share an excellent recipe using pomegranate.

1   pomegranate

1 Pound	boneless pork tenderloins, sliced into ½ inch-thick medallions
¼ tsp	Celtic Sea Salt
¼ tsp	ground black pepper
3 tsp	olive oil
½ cup	finely chopped red onion
1 cup	plain pomegranate juice
¼ cup	reduced-sodium chicken broth (or homemade broth)
1 Tbsp	honey
1 Tbsp	balsamic vinegar
3	sprigs fresh thyme

Directions: Cut the pomegranate in half through the stem. Fill a large bowl with water. Holding the pomegranate under the water, remove the seeds with your hands. Drain the seeds well. Set aside 1/3 cup. Reserve the rest for another use.

Season the medallions with the salt and pepper.

Heat 2 teaspoons of the olive oil in a skillet over medium-high heat and cook the pork until light pink in the center, 2 – 3 minutes per side. Transfer to a plate and tent loosely with foil to keep warm.

Turn the heat to medium and add the remaining 1 teaspoon oil to the skillet. Add the onion and cook, stirring, until softened, about 3 minutes. Stir in the pomegranate juice, chicken broth, honey, vinegar, and thyme. Simmer until the sauce is reduced to about ½ cup, 5 – 8 minutes.

Divide the medallions evenly among four plates and pour the sauce over each serving. Sprinkle each serving with pomegranate seeds and serve.

Fish & Shellfish:

Salmon with Pecan Pesto

Serves: 4

(recipe by Jordan S. Rubin, The Maker's Diet)

5 oz.	shelled pecans
1	3-inch sprig of rosemary
4	salmon fillets (1-1/4 to 1-1/2 pounds total)
3 oz.	cold butter, cut into ½ Tbsp pats
2 – 3	fresh jalapeño peppers, seeded and coarsely chopped
1 Tbsp	Olive Oil

Zest of ½ small lemon (or small orange), finely chopped

Celtic Sea Salt and freshly ground pepper

Preheat oven to 300 degrees Fahrenheit.

Directions: Toast pecans on a cookie sheet about 20 – 30 minutes, or until they release their aroma. Set aside to cool.

Strip rosemary leaves from stems, mince, and set aside.

Rinse salmon and pat dry. If desired, butterfly fillets with a sharp knife. Rub salmon with olive oil; season with salt and pepper. Heat heavy skillet over medium heat. Pan-fry fillets until firm to the touch.

Place toasted pecans, rosemary, butter, jalapenos, and lemon zest in a food processor. Process the blend for 5 – 8 seconds, scraping the bowl often and repeating the process two or three times until a paste (pesto) forms. Do not over-process.

Spread the pesto over cooked salmon, and serve immediately.

Mustard-Crusted Halibut

Serves: 1 – 2

(recipe by David Kirsch, The Ultimate New York Body Plan)

6 oz.	center-cut halibut steak
1 tsp	whole-grain mustard
1 tsp	chopped fresh thyme
1 Tbsp	chopped fresh oregano
1 tsp	chopped fresh rosemary
½ tsp	fresh ground black pepper
1 tsp	water
1 – 2 tsp	butter

Preheat oven to 350 degrees Fahrenheit.

Directions: In a small bowl, combine the mustard, thyme, oregano, rosemary, pepper, and water and blend well to make a paste.

Butter an ovenproof baking dish. Place halibut in the dish and spread with the mustard-herb paste. Bake for 15 to 20 minutes or until fish flakes easily with a fork.

Delightful served on a bed of baby spinach, arugula, and water chestnuts.

Spicy Mahi-Mahi and Mango Tacos

Serves: 4

3 Tbsp	fresh lime juice
3 Tbsp	fresh orange juice
1	garlic clove, chopped
2 tsp	chili powder
¼ tsp	Celtic Sea Salt
¼ tsp	ground black pepper
1/8 tsp	cayenne pepper
1 lb	Mahi-Mahi, rinsed and patted dry, cut into bite-size chunks

1	large ripe mango, peeled, pitted, and coarsely chopped (about 2 cups)
1 Tbsp	chopped red onion, rinsed and drained
¼ cup	fresh cilantro leaves, chopped
½ tsp	seeded, chopped fresh red chili
2 tsp	virgin coconut oil
4	(8) inch whole-wheat tortillas
1	ripe avocado, pitted, peeled and coarsely chopped

Lime wedges, for serving.

Directions: In medium bowl, whisk together 2 Tablespoons of the lime juice, 2 Tablespoons of the orange juice, the garlic, chili powder, salt, black pepper, and cayenne pepper. Add the fish and gently stir to coat. Let stand for at least 10 minutes, or cover and place in the refrigerator for up to 4 hours.

In the meantime, in a medium bowl, combine the mango, onion, cilantro, chili, and remaining 1 tablespoon each of the lime and orange juice. Stir gently until well combined. Set aside in the refrigerator if you are marinating the fish longer than a few minutes. Let stand at room temperature for at least 20 minutes before serving.

In a large skillet, heat the oil over medium-high heat. Add the fish and its marinade and cook for 3 to 4 minutes, turning frequently, until the fish is opaque.

While the fish cooks, wrap the tortillas in damp paper towels and microwave on high power for 30 seconds. I don't use a microwave but place the tortillas in an oven-proof dish, sprinkle with a little water, and place in the oven for 15 minutes at 350 degrees Fahrenheit.

Gently fold the avocado into the mango mixture.

Divide the fish evenly among the tortillas. Divide the mango mixture among the tacos, spooning it on top of the fish. Serve with lime wedges.

Chili-Lime Shrimp Skewers with Pineapple-Mint Salsa

Serves: 4

3 Tbsp	fresh lime juice
2 Tbsp	olive oil
1-1/4 lbs	large shrimp, peeled and deveined
1	pineapple
2 Tbsp	finely chopped red onion, rinsed and drained
¼ cup	packed fresh mint, chopped
¼ to ½ tsp	seeded and minced fresh red chili
1 tsp	chili powder
½ tsp	Celtic Sea Salt
¼ tsp	ground black pepper

Olive oil spray, for the grill or grill pan

Directions: If using a gas or charcoal grill, spray the grill with olive oil and prepare a medium-hot grill. If using a grill pan, spray it with olive oil and heat over medium-high heat.

Place (8) skewers in a pan of water; let stand for at least 20 minutes.

In a medium bowl, whisk together 2 tablespoons of the lime juice and the olive oil. Add the shrimp and stir to coat. Let stand for 15 minutes.

Use a serrated knife to cut the top off the pineapple. Cut a thin slice from the bottom and stand the pineapple upright on a cutting board. Beginning at the top, use a gentle sawing motion to cut down the length of the pineapple and remove a strip of the rough skin; try to cut deep enough that you remove most of the eyes. Repeat all the way around the pineapple until the skin is removed. Use a paring knife to remove any remaining eyes. Lay the pineapple on its side and carefully cut it crosswise into ½-inch slices.

Grill the pineapple slices just until tender, about 4 minutes per side. Transfer to a work surface. Cut the pineapple into ½ inch pieces, discarding the tough center of each slice; you should have about 4 cups. Place the pineapple in a medium bowl and add the onion, mint, chili, and remaining 1 tablespoon of lime juice. Stir gently and set aside.

Pat the shrimp dry and thread them onto the skewers. Sprinkle with the chili powder, salt, and pepper. Grill until just opaque in the center, 4 to 5 minutes, turning once. Serve with the Pineapple Mint Salsa.

Bay Scallops with Toasted Sesame Seeds
Serves: 4

2 Tbsp	olive oil
1 lb	farmed bay scallops (unless you have fresh scallops out of the ocean)
¼ tsp	Celtic Sea Salt
¼ tsp	ground pepper
1 tsp	fresh lemon juice
¼ tsp	toasted sesame oil
2 Tbsp	white or black sesame seeds, or a combination.

Lemon wedges, for serving.

Directions: In a well-seasoned cast-iron skillet big enough to hold the scallops in a single layer, heat the olive oil over medium-high heat until hot but not smoking. Add the scallops to cook, shaking the pan occasionally, until lightly browned, approx. 2 – 3 minutes.

Sprinkle the scallops with the salt and pepper, and add ¼ cup water to the pan. Cook, scraping up any browned bits, until saucy. Stir in the lemon juice and sesame oil. Transfer to a serving platter and sprinkle with the sesame seeds. Serve with lemon wedges.

CHAPTER THIRTEEN
RESTAURANT FOODS YOU'LL WANT TO AVOID & MEALS TO REPLACE THEM AT HOME

If you're like so many families, you're frequently out and about when it's mealtime and are inadvertently forced to eat in restaurants. Many restaurants serve foods that aren't really considered healthy, as they are laden with sugars, fats, artificial flavors and ingredients, all of which will make it very difficult for you to reach your weight loss goals.

As an individual concerned with health and wellness, it probably won't surprise you to find out that I am NOT a proponent of fast foods or eating in restaurants. In fact, I actually find restaurant experiences unpleasant. Why? For many reasons, including smoking (if allowed), strong perfume and/or colognes worn by other patrons that make it difficult to enjoy my meal, crying children, etc. I grew up in a home where almost every meal was prepared at home by my parents. As a matter of fact, my first "fast food" experience was when I was in the fourth grade and we met a classmate who was traveling from California to Florida at the "golden arches" to say hello and grab a quick bite to eat. Needless to say, my system was not geared for this type of food and I became ill within minutes of consuming it.

Recognizing that fast foods and restaurant foods really don't have consumer's health and wellness in mind is an important detail to consider. Acting on it will make the difference.

Below, I'm going to provide you with a few examples of foods served in some of America's most popular restaurants, so that if you find yourself in a position requiring that you choose a quick bite on the run, you can choose some of the healthier items available on the menu over less healthy options.

Now, I'm not suggesting that you eat these foods on a regular basis, as you can see for yourself that they are high in calories, fat grams, sodium, and sugar content. However, if you have no other alternative available, you can use this as a quick reference guide.

Eat This... NOT That!!!

Applebee's:
Steak & Grilled Shrimp   vs.

    390 Calories

    6 grams Saturated Fat

    1,890 mg Sodium

Grilled Shrimp and Spinach Salad

    1,040 Calories

    11 Grams Saturated Fat

    2,380 mg Sodium

Arby's:
Bacon Cheddar Roastburger   vs.

    440 Calories

    18 grams Fat: 8 Saturated; 1 Trans.

    1,427 mg. Sodium

Ultimate BLT Market Fresh Sandwich

    779 Calories

    45 grams Fat: 11 Saturated; .5 Trans

    1,571 mg. Sodium

Atlanta Bread Company:
Chicken Waldorf Sandwich   vs.

    450 Calories

    29 grams Fat: 2.5 grams Saturated

    510 mg. Sodium

Bistro Chicken Press Sandwich

    780 Calories

    41 grams Fat: 11 grams Saturated

    1,660 mg. Sodium

Baskin-Robbins:
Oreo Cookies 'n Cream Ice Cream   vs.

    365 Calories

    18 grams Fat: 10 grams Saturated

    34 grams Sugar

Oreo Outrageous Sundae

    1,130 Calories

    55 grams Fat: 27 grams Sat.

    1 gram Trans.

    120 grams Sugar

Blimpie:
Roast Beef & Provolone   vs.

    385 Calories

    12 grams Fat; 5 g saturated

    990 mg Sodium

Roast Beef & Cheddar Wrap

    684 Calories

    36 grams Fat: 12 g Saturated

    1,928 mg Sodium

Burger King:
Ham Omelet Sandwich   vs.

    290 Calories

    12 grams Fat: 4.5 g Saturated

    870 mg Sodium

Sausage & Cheese Breakfast Shots

    420 Calories

    31 grams fat: 10 g Saturated

        .5 g Trans

    910 mg Sodium

Carrabba's:
Manicotti   vs.

    640 Calories

Lasagna

    1,360 Calories

Chick-Fil-A:
Chick-fil-A Chargrilled Chicken Club   vs.   **Chicken Caesar Cool Wrap**
    380 Calories   480 Calories
    11 grams Fat: 5 g Saturated   16 grams Fat: 7 g Saturated
    1,560 mg Sodium   1,810 mg Sodium

Chili's:
Southwestern Cedar Plank Tilapia   vs.   **Southwestern Cobb Salad**
    600 Calories   1,080 Calories
    27 grams Fat: 4 g Saturated   71 grams fat: 16 g Saturated
    1,820 mg Sodium   2.650 mg Sodium

Dairy Queen:
Hot Fudge Sundae   vs.   **Hot Fudge Malt**
    300 Calories   700 Calories
    10 grams Fat: 7 g Saturated   23 grams Fat: 16 g Saturated/
                                         1 g Trans.
    37 grams Sugar   85 grams Sugar

Denny's:
Top Sirloin Steak & Fried Eggs   vs.   **Heartland Scramble**
    420 Calories   1,150 Calories
    21 grams Fat: 6 g Saturated   66 grams Fat: 20 g Saturated/
             .5 Trans.   .5 g Trans.
    920 mg Sodium   2,800 mg. Sodium

iHop:
Spinach, Mushroom & Tomato Omelette vs.   **Garden Omelette**
    330 Calories   1,030 Calories
    7 grams Fat: 3 g Saturated   20.5 grams Saturated Fat
    660 mg Sodium   1,230 mg Sodium

Jamba Juice:
Berry Fulfilling   vs.   **Banana Berry**
    270 Calories   400 Calories
    1 gram Fat   1.5 grams Fat
    45 grams Sugar   82 grams Sugar

Long John Silver's
Grilled Pacific Salmon   vs.

249 Calories
8 grams Fat: 1.5 g Saturated
440 mg Sodium

Fish Sandwich

470 Calories
27 grams Fat: 5 g Saturated/
4.5 g Trans
1,210 mg Sodium

McDonalds
McDouble   vs.

390 Calories
19 grams Fat: 8 g Saturated/1 g Trans
920 mg Sodium

Grilled Chicken Club Sandwich

530 Calories
17 grams Fat: 6 g Saturated
1,210 mg Sodium

Olive Garden
Ravioli di Portobello   vs.

450 Calories
19 grams Fat: 11 g Saturated
970 mg Sodium

Manicotti Formaggio

880 Calories
33 grams Fat: 18 g Saturated
2,100 mg Sodium

On the Border
Pico Shrimp Tacos   vs.

490 Calories
5 grams Fat: 1 g Saturated
1,650 mg Sodium

Grilled Mahi Mahi Fish Tacos

1,200 Calories
61 grams Fat: 13 g Saturated
3,080 mg Sodium

Outback
Grilled Chicken & Swiss Sandwich   vs.

696 Calories
33 grams Fat: 10 g Saturated
1,323 mg Sodium

Alice Springs Chicken

1,679 Calories
115 grams fat: 53 g Saturated
2,686 mg Sodium

Panda Express
Pineapple Chicken and Broccoli Beef   vs.

380 Calories
16 grams Fat: 3.5 g Saturated
1,430 mg Sodium

Orange Chicken

820 Calories
20 grams Fat: 3.5 g Saturated
840 mg Sodium

Papa John's
Thin Crust BBQ Chicken & Bacon Pizza, 14"   vs.

540 Calories
26 grams Fat: 7 g Saturated
1,500 mg Sodium

Pan Crust Hawaiian BBQ Chicken Pizza, 12"

880 Calories
44 grams fat: 14 g Saturated
1,880 mg Sodium

Popeye's

Spicy Chicken Legs vs. **Spicy Chicken Thigh**

320 Calories

14 grams Fat: 6 g Saturated

1,030 mg Sodium

620 Calories

43 grams Fat: 14 g Saturated/ .5 Trans.

1,200 mg Sodium

Quiznos

Roadhouse Steak Sammie vs. **Prime Rib Cheesesteak Sub**

380 Calories

12 grams Fat: 3 g Saturated

1,335 mg Sodium

670 Calories

41 grams fat: 10 g Saturated/1 g Tran

1,085 mg Sodium

Red Lobster

Live Maine Lobster (1-1/4 lbs) vs. **Chef's Signature Lobster & Shrimp Pasta**

475 Calories

19 grams Fat: 4 g Saturated

1,680 mg Sodium

1,020 Calories

50 g Fat: 22 g Saturated

2,180 mg Sodium

Ruby Tuesday

Turkey Burger Wrap vs. **Turkey Minis**

551 Calories

19 grams Fat

44 g Carbohydrates

1,058 Calories

58 grams Fat

79 g Carbohydrates

Smoothie King

Blueberry Heaven vs. **Skinny Cranberry Supreme**

325 Calories

1 gram Fat

64 grams Sugar

454 Calories

1 gram Fat

73 grams Sugar

Starbucks

Turkey Cranberry Pesto vs. **Tarragon Chicken Salad Sandwich**

480 Calories

19 grams Fat: 2 g Saturated

26 grams Sugar

990 mg Sodium

740 Calories

12 grams Fat: 2 g Saturated

73 grams Sugar

1,335 mg Sodium

Subway

Steak and Cheese vs. **Meatball Marinara**

    390 Calories   580 Calories

    10 grams Fat: 4.5 g Saturated   23 grams Fat: 9 g Saturated

    1,670 mg Sodium   1,660 mg Sodium

Taco Bell

Fresco Crunch Beef Tacos vs. **Chipotle Steak Fully Loaded Salad**

    450 Calories   950 Calories

    21 grams Fat: 7.5 g Saturated   59 grams fat: 11 g Saturated/1 g Tran

    750 mg Sodium   1,760 mg Sodium

Wendy's

Spicy Chicken Fillet Sandwich vs. **Chicken Club Sandwich**

    440 Calories   550 Calories

    16 grams Fat: 3 g Saturated   26 grams Fat: 8 g Saturated

    1,200 mg Sodium   1,290 mg Sodium

It isn't always wise to assume that what you think is the healthiest choice on the menu actually is the healthiest. Using this chart, and reading the calorie, fat, and sodium information often provided, will help you make better choices when dining out.

CHAPTER FOURTEEN
TIPS TO REMEMBER AT MEALTIME

Losing weight isn't always a walk in the park. In fact, it can be quite difficult if you are operating on a set of beliefs that doesn't quite hold water. Knowing the facts and then incorporating them into your lifestyle will help you achieve your weight loss goals in a timelier manner.

Avoiding the hype and promotions for a "quick diet" or "lose weight fast" scheme is often difficult, but definitely worth resisting. Often, these diets, or "quick fixes," will throw your metabolism off, making it much more difficult to get back on track.

The best method, and safest, is to carefully watch what you eat and how much. Modifying your eating habits along with incorporating a fitness program into your life will provide you the better and long-lasting results that you desire.

Tips of the Trade:

> **Measure your portions.** This tip COULD make all of the difference in the world when it comes to losing weight or eating portions that will assist you in maintaining your weight. While I am a healthy eater, I wasn't paying attention to the size of my portions. Without thinking I'd serve my plate using the same portions that I'd serve my growing teenage sons, not giving any consideration that a healthy and recommended serving of rice was 1/2 cup (120 calories). I was easily eating three times that. If you are still hungry after eating what's on your plate and desire seconds, it's wiser to opt for a serving of vegetables or a salad. A good rule of thumb when serving your meal is that one half of the plate should be vegetables, one fourth proteins, one fourth starches.

> Measure while cooking too! I was extremely generous with the olive oil when roasting vegetables, for example. Instead of using the amount recommended, I'll bet I was using up to 1/4 cup (475 calories) or more when I could have gotten by with half that amount.

> **Sit down to eat meals and snacks.** All meals should be eaten at the table (or counter) while sitting. Standing in front of the refrigerator, at the vending machine, or in front of the

television is no way to eat – in fact, you'll be better able to monitor what and how much you're eating if you are sitting and it is in front of you on a plate

Stop eating your kids' leftovers. If they don't eat it and you aren't willing to save it for them to eat later, toss it. A quarter of a ham and cheese here, ½ cup of leftover macaroni and cheese there - it all adds up. You've heard the saying, "A minute on the lips – A lifetime on the hips" – it's true!!! Is it worth it?

Keep a food log and take advantage of online calorie counters. If you use the food charts provided, you'll be quite safe at monitoring your daily caloric intake. Remember, eliminating calories can be risky – especially if you don't eat enough of them for your daily maintenance. I should know. I worked out with a personal trainer for several years and wasn't consuming enough calories. My body weight remained the same and I never lost the pudge around the midsection. There are many calorie-counters available, however, one that is quick and easy (and free) is: www.thecaloriecounter.com. This website is a comprehensive database of all foods. If you have an iPhone, you can also download and use the free application called Lose It!

Bump up your exercise to create a calorie deficit. Although I've not discussed exercise thus far, it is imperative that you engage in some form of it daily in order to stay fit, help you lose weight, build muscle, and improve your cardiovascular health. Having said you need to exercise, creating a calorie deficit is a great tool to assist you in losing weight – as long as your deficit is from exercise and not starvation. For example, just an extra 30 minutes of walking will burn approximately 120 calories. Completed first thing in the morning while it is still comfortable outside, you'll also boost your metabolism for the day!

Easy food substitutions (to reduce calories) that have worked for me:

- Drink your coffee black and save as much as 75 calories per coffee cup from dropping cream and sugar, or eliminate coffee and caffeine altogether and drink water with lemon (great for heart health and reducing blood pressure naturally).

- Ditch the mayo (100 calories per tablespoon) on your lunchtime sandwich. If you just cannot go without, try using light mayo (50 calories per tablespoon); fat free mayo, although I don't recommend using fat-free anything (11 calories per tablespoon); or mustard (20 calories per tablespoon) and save up to 90 calories. Take the top piece of bread off the sandwich and save another 70 calories, or use a whole-grain wrap and save more.

- You can still have chips, but make them baked (56 calories for ten) vs. regular fried (120 calories). Pita chips are an excellent choice and they use sea salt vs. table salt.

- Choose the right salad dressing. Ranch dressing is 148 calories for 2 tablespoons, while a fat free Italian has 14 calories for the same serving size. A squeeze of fresh lemon with the tiniest drizzle of olive oil is a delicious option and the one that I'd recommend.

CHAPTER FIFTEEN
EXERCISE… IT ISN'T JUST FOR JOCKS

I've seen the fancy commercials, "Lose weight without exercising," "Lose weight without modifying your habits," and I'm sure you have too. But, have you ever seen anyone with an incredible body that has eliminated all forms of exercise and diet? I'd guess you probably have not – and why? Simply put: because a nice physique does not exist in reality without some form of exercise to tone and shape. Anyone who tells you otherwise is pulling the wool over your eyes and convincing you to believe in something that couldn't be farther from the truth.

Some form of exercise is required for your body to feel and look better, both inside and out. With an increase of cardiovascular disease on the horizon, you should welcome the opportunity to exercise your heart and reduce the risk of falling victim to something so preventable. Sitting on your behind, falling for the latest contraption and gadget promising you that you won't have to do anything other than to "strap this on" or "pop this pill" will leave you susceptible to many forms of illness. The truth is: If you don't use it – you lose it! I'm talking about muscles.

Exercise, in one form or another, is something that everyone must participate in order to make their weight loss goals a reality. Now, this doesn't mean that you must join a gym, running club, or take up mountain climbing. What it does mean is that you must do something that will increase your heart rate and strengthen and tone your muscles. So what advice can I offer you on this subject? Plenty, but I'll keep it brief.

Exercise 101:

Exercise isn't for everyone – but it should be. Not only does it improve cardiovascular health, but it builds, strengthens, and tones our muscles. It increases one's stamina, decreases blood pressure (along with proper nutrition and diet), and keeps the mind young and sharp. You might not believe it, but it also allows one's skin to radiate a youthful appearance even when you're fifty or sixty. Exercise is truly one of life's best gifts, for without it life expectancy is reduced.

You're probably making the statement, "Here we go - another weight loss plan that suggests I get my behind into the gym." The good news is I'm not recommending you sign a contract to join a gym or club that will cost you money. In fact, I'm going to suggest a few things that won't cost you a dime. I've spent many hours in the gym, and although the results were plenty, and costly, I could have accomplished the same at home.

So, without further ado, let me reintroduce you to a few exercise suggestions that you can do anywhere, with little or no equipment, and best of all, you can do with a loved one, friend, or family pet, or by yourself… Walking!!!

Exercise Tips & Suggestions:

Think back to a time when you were a mere child and you didn't even know what a gym or gym equipment was. Like so many, you were probably in the best shape of your life. By simply engaging in daily physical activities such as playing dodge ball, jumping rope, hula hoop, jumping on a trampoline, or climbing a tree your body was strong, lean, and I'll bet something you wish you could recapture today. You can, almost, given that you'll have to consider the changes that your body has experienced throughout the years.

If you'll recall from an earlier chapter, there are some changes that our bodies have experienced that cannot be undone. For instance, I've had two healthy baby boys that I couldn't be more proud of; unfortunately, they were big for my small stature. As a result, my hips (pelvic region) widened and I now have stretch marks across my stomach and hips. In terms of body changes, this is the nature of the birthing game. Although I'd love to reclaim my perfect skin and more narrow hips, I cannot. I simply have to work with what I've been left to perfect as best I can. You, too, may have experienced changes that you cannot modify to a previous state, but you can improve it.

When beginning any fitness program, you'll always want to check with your primary care physician to ensure that it is safe for you and takes into account any and all preexisting conditions that you may have. For instance, if you have high blood pressure or you're diabetic, your doctor may want you to take it easy when launching an exercise program to determine any special precautions that may need to be considered. Remember, you're modifying your lifestyle and don't want to shock your system unnecessarily.

Tips & Suggestions:

a) A good rule of thumb to consider when choosing an exercise program is to choose something that you enjoy!!! Case in point: If you don't enjoy it, you won't do it! A perfect example would be someone who loves to jog; they'll enjoy this activity daily while others may hate it. If you cannot stand the thought of doing it – trust me when I say you won't do it. Choose something that you enjoy. I enjoy going for walks. It provides me a time to be alone, clear my head, and prepare for my day. Because I enjoy it, I make time to do it daily – sometimes more than once a day. Keep in mind that with any exercise program, you don't have to cram it all in at once. You can spread your chosen activities out over a day, week, or month. I walk twice a day – once in the morning before it becomes hot and muggy (I live in Georgia), and once in the evening when the sun has gone down and I can unwind for the day. Note: Walking is considered by most healthcare professionals to be one of the healthiest methods of exercise for building strength and stamina, and reducing weight. It puts less stress on your joints (than running), allows you to increase and decrease one's heart rate by simply speeding up or slowing down, and can be modified by simply choosing a different terrain.

b) Choose multiple activities that will allow you some variety. Variety is the spice of life, and this couldn't come into play more than when talking about exercise. Exercise can get boring if you do the same thing day in and day out. Spice it up! Choose two or three different activities that you can enjoy and mix it up. I enjoy walking, as noted above, but I also like to swim, ride my bike, dance, strengthen my mind, body, and soul via yoga and pilates, and workout with weights. Lucky for me, I can do all of these at home and with very little equipment. I simply alternate my activities so that I am always engaging in something different. You can do this too, by simply choosing a few things that you enjoy and then incorporating them into your daily routine.

c) Invite a friend to participate along with you. If you are the type who will "put off today what you can do tomorrow," you'll find it difficult to change your lifestyle and/or your body. You may have to schedule your activities with someone who will help hold you accountable. Case in point: Having a gym membership doesn't mean that you'll actually go to the gym. Over the years I found this to be true of so many people. Scheduling an appointment to work out with a trainer will increase the likelihood that you go, as you'll not only be impacting his/her schedule, but there is also a monetary fee associated with training. Including another individual in your routine may teach you to be more dependable in terms of keeping your scheduled workout appointment(s), and it will probably increase accountability, as you will undoubtedly learn more about the value of the dollar lost. Enjoying an activity with another will allow you to experience a social environment/aspect, which will more than likely increase the enjoyment of your participation.

d) Use a calendar to assist you in scheduling your exercise/activities. By calendaring your time, you can make certain that you've allocated a portion of each day to getting the physical exercise that your body needs to be healthy. More often than not you'll hear individuals say, "I just didn't have time," or "I'm so busy," when asked if they were able to do this and/or that during the course of the day. Eliminate excuses by making time for yourself – aren't you worth it?

e) With any exercise regime, you should include strength training along with cardiovascular exercise. This doesn't mean that you need to rush out and purchase a gym set, or even dumbbells. Strength training can be accomplished using a variety of easily accessible items right at home. For instance, if you shop for groceries you can use a gallon of milk; a bag of sugar or flour; or even a bag of potatoes to build strength in your upper body. Instead of allowing the grocer to take your groceries to the car and unload them for you, do it yourself. If you've got stairs at home, you can build strength in your legs by walking up and down them a couple of times per day; to increase your endurance and provide more weight, carry a phone book, basket of laundry, or even use simple strap-on ankle weights. Most individuals own a VCR or DVD player, and if you have children you've probably got some type of gaming system such as Xbox or Wii. Each of these electronic(s) will have training/exercise activities that you can enjoy by simply slipping in the disc and pressing play. Of course, you have to participate – simply watching the screen while sitting on your behind will not melt away the pounds or provide you the heart-healthy exercise that you need.

f) Keep a journal of your activities so that you can see the differences in your physical appearance, and your emotional welfare too. I've included both a before and after space for you to attach a photo. There is nothing more motivating than to see the differences that you're making in your life. As you'll recall, I asked you to include a sentence or description of how you hope to see yourself in three, six, and nine months from the date you begin your lifestyle makeover. Please complete this section, as it is extremely important for your overall success. You'll also see spaces for your body measurements that I hope you'll use, as this can be a very motivating tool as well.

List of Exercises: Cardiovascular Activities
a) **Walking**
b) **Jogging**
c) **Swimming**
d) **Hula Hoop**
e) **Jump Rope**
f) **Mini-Trampoline/Trampoline**
g) **Cycling**
h) **Dancing or Dance Class (Ballet; Tap; Jazz; Modern)**
i) **Tennis**
j) **Basketball**
k) **Tetherball**
l) **Boxing**
m) **Exercise Class – (Step; Martial Arts; Spin; Aerobics; Belly Dancing)**
n) **Soccer**
o) **Volleyball**
p) **Table Tennis**
q) **Physical Fitness Games (Xbox, Wii)**
r) **Water Aerobics**
s) **Roller Skating**
t) **Ice Skating**
u) **Snow Skiing (Cross Country)**
v) **Water Skiing**
w) **Rowing**
x) **Skipping**
y) **Circuit Training**
z) **Stepper**

List of Exercises: Strength Training Activities
   a) Weight Training
   b) Yoga
   c) Pilates
   d) Resistance Band Exercises
   e) Gymnastics
   f) Triathlon Training
   g) Rock Climbing
   h) Exercise Ball
   i) Hockey
   j) Baseball
   k) Golf
   l) Snow Skiing
   m) Throwing

   n) Calisthenics: Arms

      1. Push-ups
      2. Knee push-ups
      3. Wall push-ups
      4. One-armed push-ups
      5. Diamond push-ups
      6. Dive bomber push-ups
      7. Explosive push-ups
      8. Incline push-ups (use a step or foot stool for arms)
      9. Decline push-ups (place feet on step or stool)
      10. Handstand push-ups
      11. Tricep dips (couch or chair for support)
      12. Suspended tricep dips with legs up on chairs
      13. Pull ups
      14. Chin ups
      15. Bar Hang (hold position as attempt a pull-up)

   o) Abdominals & Obliques

      16. Sit-ups
      17. V-situps
      18. Full boat pose (Yoga)
      19. Rope climbing sit ups
      20. Incline sit ups
      21. Crunches
      22. Reverse crunches
      23. Rope climbing crunches
      24. Oblique twists
      25. Double crunches (both upper and lower body compressed)

26. Single leg crunches (legs up 90 degrees, bring leg across body)
27. Extended arms overhead abdominal curls
28. Butterfly leg abdominal curl
29. Extended leg pendulum drop
30. 90 degree leg scissors
31. Low legged scissors
32. Flutter kicks
33. Bent knee side-to-side twists
34. Side plank upper body twists
35. Cross legged abdominal lifter
36. Bridge
37. Standing side curls
38. Plank
39. Side plank
40. The one hundred (Pilates)

p) Back

41. Trunk lifts
42. Tummy lying Leg lifts
43. Alternating SuperMan arm/leg lifts
44. Combined trunk/leg extensions
45. Rotating trunk extensions
46. Bow poses (Yoga)
47. Cobra poses (Yoga)
48. The saw (Pilates)

q) Lower Body

49. Squats
50. Half squats
51. Wall squats
52. Sumo squats
53. Plie squats
54. One legged squats
55. Squat kicks
56. Chair pose 1 (Yoga)
57. Lunges
58. Side lunges
59. Reverse lunges
60. Walking lunges
61. Jumping lunges
62. Step up lunges
63. Lunging kicks

64. Star jumps
65. Wall jumps
66. Forward jumps
67. One-legged hop
68. Forward kicks
69. Back-kicks
70. Side-kicks
71. Roundhouse kicks
72. Calf raises
73. One-legged calf raises
74. One-legged dead lifts
75. Reverse hip lifts
76. Dirty dogs (side knee lifts/on all fours)
77. Downward facing dogs (form body into an A frame position)
78. Kneeling rear straight leg lifts
79. Kneeling rear bent leg lifts
80. Kneeling bent leg inward press (knee pressed toward body's opposite calf)
81. Lying side leg raises
82. Standing side leg raises
83. Standing rear leg lifts
84. Side lying bottom leg raises
85. Side lying dual leg lifts
86. Side plank
87. Lying leg circles
88. Lying single leg circles

Well, there you have it. Over 100 exercises that you can do at home to build, strengthen, tone, and improve your heart's health through both strength training exercises and cardiovascular activities. By incorporating these into your daily routine, if only a few a day, you'll begin to see noticeable differences in your overall health and wellness and physique.

What are you waiting for? Let's get started today!!!

CHAPTER SIXTEEN
TOXINS IN YOUR HOME

In addition to the information that I've researched and provided you regarding diet, exercise, and the many foods that you'll want to avoid as they can convert into sugar, store in your body as fat, and throw off your metabolic system, I wanted to include a special article that I wrote for and published on www.childrentopics.com about toxins that can be found in just about any home. Why? Because the information contained within will explain how toxins found in everyday consumable products can actually be hurting us instead of keeping us healthy. Please take the time to read, enjoy, and learn from the article. Trust me, you'll be glad you did.

Our Toxic World (Harmful Chemicals found in Everyday Products)

Is your home a chemical danger zone? If you're like most families, a large number of products that you use every day for cleaning your home, personal hygiene, and even some pharmaceuticals can actually contain harmful toxins and pose hazards to your health. In fact, most families will only need to look as far as their kitchen cabinets to uncover a staggering amount of products containing harmful toxins.

Perhaps you've never really given it much thought until you see something on a news broadcast or hear a friend, neighbor, or relative talking about someone who is stricken by the loss resulting from chemical ingestion, burn, or exposure. It usually takes something substantial to make us wake up and take the necessary steps to eliminate the chances of it happening to us or our loved ones.

From laundry detergents and air fresheners, to baby shampoos and toothpastes, you should know the potential dangers of the products that you bring into your home and how to safeguard your children, pets, and even yourself from the toxins that you probably don't even know you have within your cabinets.

In general, I believe that most of us can determine which chemicals are harmful based upon the smell or even the labeling - **KEEP OUT OF REACH OF CHILDREN** being a pretty good clue. What about those products and chemicals that we use daily which aren't labeled as dangerous and actually are? Today we are bombarded with information on how toxic chemicals, pollution, and

212 • Randa Lee Roberts

other threats are having a devastating impact on our environment; however, very little is published or made available to families as it relates to the negative effects consumable products have on our personal environment(s) a.k.a., "our bodies."

Perhaps our society is just too comfortable with the easy-clean, easy-care disposable lifestyles that we've nestled ourselves into to pay attention or really provide any thought to what the exposures are capable of doing to us. This, of course, is why I ask the question, "Aren't you concerned with the fact that your body burden of toxic chemicals contains lead, mercury, flame retardants, Bisphenol A (BPA), DDT, PCBs, and many more? (For more on Bisphenol A, check out my article entitled, "The Harmful Effects of BPA" at www.childrentopics.com.) I believe that if parents and caregivers knew just how many serious illnesses and deaths were directly related to the chemicals that we are exposed to on a daily basis, they'd be more likely to heed the warnings that are out there, perhaps not as boldly as McDonald's as they should be in an effort to gain the attention of consumers. So, it is my goal today to make you a healthier consumer by educating you. After all, the healthiest consumer is an educated one!

There are many companies that advertise their products as organic, eco-friendly, and toxin-free. You've heard the phrase used in real estate, "Buyer Beware?" Well, it should also be applied to everyday products that we purchase with the intention of using at home with and on our children, ourselves, AND our pets. Purchase products that are truly safer, healthier, and oftentimes more economical due to the concentrated formulas utilized to reduce packaging that will either ultimately end up in a landfill, should you not recycle, or be reused within your home to cut down on waste. Fact: If every household in North America used concentrated products such as EcoSense TM products INSTEAD of grocery store brands, in 10 years we would save almost 7 billion pounds of plastic. If the plastic saved were converted into plastic laundry baskets, it would circle the earth 71 times!!!

I bet you are unaware of the **United States of America Federal Code of Regulations** that exempts manufacturers from providing the entire contents of products contained in products on the labeling IF used for personal, family, or household care. **(USA FCR: Section 1910.1200C, Title 29, Section 1500.82 2Q1A)**. This loophole in labeling practices allows manufacturers to use harmful chemicals and toxins within consumable products that actually have been linked to various health-related issues such as cancer, diabetes, leukemia, etc. Perhaps you're also unaware of the National Safety Council's finding that more children under the age of four die due to accidental household poisonings than the number of reported deaths resulting from accidental shootings within the home.

The results from studies that have been conducted are quite shocking. In fact, The **Environmental Protection Agency** (with whom I was once employed) released the results from a study indicating that toxic chemicals in household cleaners are three times more likely to cause cancer than outdoor air pollution, and they also stated that indoor air pollution can be 3 to 70 times higher than outdoor air pollution. With information such as these findings, it would seem consumers would want to take a stand.

In a study on personal care products such as shampoos, deodorants, toothpastes, lotions, body washes/soaps, hairspray, etc., a shocking 2,983 chemicals were analyzed and provided the following results:

- 884   were toxic
- 145   can result in tumors
- 218   were linked to reproductive complications
- 778   cause acute toxicity
- 314   can result in biological mutations
- 376   can lead to skin and eye irritations

(Source: United States House of Representatives Report through NIOSH, 1989)

Of the chemicals analyzed, it was determined that 90% of the poisonings occurred via inhalation and skin absorption, while 10% of the household poisonings were a result of ingestion. The Consumer Protection Agency reported that 150 chemicals found within the home have been directly linked to allergies, birth defects, cancer, and psychological disorders. Shockingly, chemicals have replaced bacteria and viruses as the main threat to our health, and in fact, diseases that used to occur later in life are now much more prevalent at younger ages. For instance, a 28% increase in childhood cancer has been noted since the addition of pesticides into household products, i.e., food, cotton, etc. Additionally, cancer is now the #2 killer of children, second to accidental poisonings.

<u>Chlorine Bleach:</u>
Parents, teachers, caregivers, custodians, medical staff, and others are very conscientious about disinfecting their homes and children's toys, especially if multiple children and/or adults will be present and/or using them. So, naturally, of particular concern to me as a mother and former

educator is household bleach. Parents use it for many purposes: bleaching diapers and using it in everyday laundry; to rid certain spaces of mold and mildew; even to clean the tile within kitchens and bathrooms. Teachers and medical facilities use it to disinfect toys, surfaces, etc, Bleaches, which claim to disinfect, are classified as pesticides under the Federal Hazardous Substances Act. Accidents happen, especially when bleach is inadvertently mixed with other chemicals, most notably, ammonia. In fact, it produces a toxic chloramines gas that can cause severe coughing, loss of voice, a burning sensation, the feeling of being suffocated, and even death. This happened to me in college without my having any idea of the dangers of mixing chemicals when cleaning my college dormitory bathroom. Perhaps, having had the knowledge, I could have avoided a very painful and embarrassing situation. (Source: Guide to Hazardous Products Around the Home, Household Hazardous Waste Project, 1989).

Formaldehyde:

Another highly toxic substance, and one of the most common indoor air pollutants, is formaldehyde. Would you believe it is used in more products than I can list for your review? Formaldehyde is suspected as one of the highest cancer-causing agents with which we unknowingly come into contact. It is an irritant to eyes, nose, throat, and lungs, and contact with the chemical agent can result in varying reactions including, but not limited to, skin irritations, ear infections, headaches, depression, joint pain, dizziness, nausea, sleep disturbances, vomiting, and fatigue. You're probably asking yourself right now, "I read the labels of the products that I purchase, so why don't I see it listed?" Well, that's simple; manufacturers can use over 30 different trade names for formaldehyde. Below are just a few:

- Formalin
- Quaternium-15 (formaldehyde-releasing agent)
- Methanal
- Methyl Aldehyde
- Methylene Oxide
- Oxymethylene
- Bfv*
- Fannoform*
- Formol*
- Fyde*
- Karsan*

- Methaldehyde
- Formalith*
- Methylene Glycol - very commonly used
- Ivalon*
- Oxomethane*
- Formalin 40
- Formic Aldehyde
- Hoch
- Paraform
- Lysoform*
- Morbocid
- Trioxane
- Polyoxmethylene

* denotes a trade name

Upon concluding the research for this article, I reviewed the labels on a random selection of products found in my sons' bathrooms, the laundry room, and kitchen (cleaning agents and chemicals), as well as in a variety of locations within and around our home. You'd be surprised at the number of products and objects that you have that contain these harmful ingredients. A short list includes: off-gasses (evaporations) from seat cushions on couches, chairs; particleboard used in some kitchens, closets and storage areas; adhesives used to manufacture most of the inexpensive wood-based products, carpets, and carpet padding.

For additional information on formaldehyde, please visit http://www.epa.gov/iaq/formalde.html

The harmful chemical agents found within and around our homes and workplaces doesn't stop there. The following list of chemicals can be found under your roof and may surprise you:

- **Radon.** According to the United States Surgeon General, the second-leading cause of lung cancer in the USA is attributed to this natural radioactive gas that seeps into the homes through cracks in the basement, crawlspace, or foundation. It is also found in well water. Radon is invisible and enters the body via airways. (My grandmother, who lived a clean life free of alcohol, tobacco, and other harmful chemicals was diagnosed with and died from cancer. When placing her home on the market, it was discovered that her home contained three times the safe level of radon inside. She lived alone and rarely allowed the home to "air out." Was this the cause of her cancer and untimely death – perhaps.)

- **Lead**. Commonly found in paint used in older homes, old plumbing, and soil near highways and busy roads, it is associated with neurological and kidney damage, high blood pressure, disrupted blood cell production, and reproductive problems. Levels once considered acceptable are now known contributors to learning disabilities and behavioral problems.

- **Carbon Monoxide** kills as estimated 660 Americans per year. It's invisible, so don't look for exhaust fumes in the attached garage to be the culprit. The primary contributor is an unserviced furnace burning propane, butane, and/or oil.

- **Arsenic.** What? Yes, this toxin is still found in many household pesticides and is used as a wood preservative. Low levels of inorganic arsenic can be linked to lung cancer according to the CDC (Centers for Disease Control).

- **Vinyl Chloride** is something that car buyers actually get excited about - what is it? It is the source of the "new car" smell. The plastic interior found in cars, playpens, and other objects with the same pleather interior produces vapors that are known carcinogens. Just like water sitting in PVC pipes overnight may create a toxic tea. Extensive exposure can cause severe liver damage and ballooning of the fingertips.

- **Hydrofluoric acid**. Found in many household rust removers, it can result in intense pain and damage to tissues and bone if protective wear isn't used.

Although the list just presented can be extremely dangerous, leading to serious illness and death, those toxins pale in comparison to the next list of volatile organic compounds, a.k.a., VOCs. VOCs include hundreds of natural and man-made, carbon-based agents. They are known to interact with other carbon-based compounds, and evaporate easily, which makes them ideal solvents. VOCs can also be found in many household disinfectants and pesticides, too.

Solvents. There are many solvents that can be found in just as many products. You'll be able to identify them by the following:

- **Benzene**
- **Methyl**
- **Ethyl**
- **Ketone**

Then there are the first cousins to this group, which you'll find on labels, such as:

- **Toluene**
- **Xylene**
- **1,1,1-trichloroethane**
- **Trichloroethylene**

Each chemical referenced above are known carcinogens and can be found in products such as lotions, deodorants, etc.

Disinfectants. Phenols, which include biphenyl, phenolics, and the preservative Pentachloraphenol, are found in disinfectants, antiseptics, perfumes, mouthwashes, glues, and air fresheners.

Pesticides. Obviously there are many, but chlordane, aldrin, and dieldrin (all of which have been banned for nearly two decades) continue to show up airborne in older homes.

Avoid being a statistical figure on the CDC's tracking list. As an adult with the capability of reading labels (take a magnifying glass), make certain that the chemicals, foods, and products that you use within and around your home don't pose threats to you and your family. Ingredient awareness, although time consuming, is definitely worth the time spent reading if it means more time living a healthy and productive life.

Replacing toxic agents with non-toxic, eco-friendly alternatives will reduce the side effects and often-debilitating illnesses that we suffer without even realizing where or how we've been exposed. Knowing that each of the agents referenced in this article are prevalent in most household products, even our foods and drinks, should influence us to shop more wisely.

What if you could replace the toxic products found within your home with products that are safer for your family, home, and for the earth? Would you do it? What if you discovered that products containing NO chlorine bleach, ammonia, aerosols, or formaldehyde were available at a fraction of the cost, and could be delivered right to your door? What if those same household products were exceptionally effective and derived from natural ingredients with NO abrasives and were pH-balanced (non-alkaline). And, what if you were able to receive each of the products outlined above in super-concentrated formulas with NO fillers or phosphates? Would you make the switch? The good news is that everything I just mentioned is available through an established wellness company that built its company on the premise that products that we use every day should be safe for you, your home, and the environment. If you're interested and want more information, please visit me at https://www.facebook.com/Living-Earth-Friendly-147564288605012/.

For practical ideas on reducing your family's risk from harmful chemicals, you can visit your local library or bookstore to consult the following books: *Living Healthy in a Toxic World*, by David Steinman and R. Michael Wisner; *Toxins A - Z: A Guide to Everyday Pollution Hazards*, by John Harte, Cheryl Holdren, Richard Schneider, and Christine Shirley.

BIBLIOGRAPHY

Batmanghelidj, F. (1992). *Your Body's Many Cries for Water*. Vienna, VA: Global Health Solutions, Inc.

Chek, Paul (2004). *How to Eat, Move and Be Healthy*. San Diego, CA: C.H.E.K. Institute

Cruise, Jorge (2009). *The Belly Fat Cure*. Carlsbad, CA: Hay House.

Dane, Elizabeth Dr. (date unknown). *Learn How You Can Thrive*. www.elizabethdane.com/?page_id=38, accessed May 2011.

Daniel, Kaayla T. (2005). *The Whole Soy Story: The Dark Side of America's Favorite Health Food*. Washington, DC: New Trends.

De Los Rios, Isabel (2009). The Diet Solution – Start Eating & Start Living, 3rd edition. Florham Park, NJ: Isabel De Los Rios.

Fallon, Sally, with Mary G. Enig (2001). *Nourishing Traditions: The Cookbook that Challenges Politically Correct Nutrition and the Diet Dictocrats*, 2nd edition. Washington, DC: New Trends.

FDA/CFSAN Federal Register 63 FR 16417 April 3, 1998 – Final Rule: Sucralose

B.K.S. Iyengar . (2007). *Yoga: The Path to Holistic Health*, Canada: Dorling Kindersley.

Kirsch, David (2005). *The Ultimate New York Body Plan*. New York, NY: McGraw-Hill.

Mercola, Joseph (2005). *Dr. Mercola's Total Health Program: The Proven Plan to Prevent Disease and Premature Aging, Optimize Weight, and Live Longer*. Schaumburg, IL: Joseph Mercola. Available from www.mercola.com/forms/total_health_book.ntm, accessed June 2008.

Michaels, Jillian. (2010). *Master Your Metabolism Cookbook*. New York, NY: Random House.

Ophardt, Charles E. (2003). *Sucralose or Splenda*. Elmhurst, IL. Available at www.elmhurst.edu/~chm/vchembook/549sucralose.html, accessed February 2010.

Regenerative Nutrition (date unknown). *Celtic Ocean Sea Salt*. www.regenerativenutrition.com/content.asp?id=30, accessed March 2011.

Rubin, Jordan S. (2004). *The Maker's Diet*. Lake Mary, FL: Siloam.

The Courier Post, Cherry Hill, N.J., August 15, 2004, Shawn Rhea

Wolcott, William, and Trish Fahey (2000). *The Metabolic Typing Diet*, New York, NY: Doubleday.

Zinczenko, David, with Matt Goulding (2010). *Eat This Not That*. Emmaus, PA: Rodale, Inc.

ABOUT THE AUTHOR

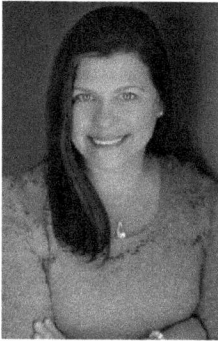

Randa Lee Roberts is the mother of two young men who have been her inspiration since their births. Committed to helping others, she launched a parenting website in January 2010, for which she both researches and writes about many different family and child growth-related issues. Originally from the small town of Monticello, Florida, she now lives outside of Atlanta, Georgia. She attended both Florida State University and the University of Florida, where she received multiple degrees and certifications in Early Childhood Education, Elementary Education, Educational Leadership and policy with Minors in Psychology and Health Education. She attended the University of West Georgia, where she obtained additional certifications in Educational Leadership.

While in attendance at F.S.U., she continued her lifelong quest for physical health and fitness and began sharing her knowledge with others through various business/job ventures. She became a health instructor for a local health and wellness clinic, while coaching youth soccer for the Y.M.C.A. Desiring to assist those unable to join a gym, she provided a mobile personal training service, and offered both individualized and group training sessions of calisthenics and cardiovascular exercise programs for employees with the State of Florida. Although never intending to compete, she continued her own personal body building under the instruction of Richard Baldwin, former Mr. Florida, Mr. Northern Hemisphere, Mr. USA, Mr. America-MW, NPC National Champion-MW, and 1st Runner-up IFBB Mr. Universe, while learning everything she could about proper diet and nutrition.

As a full-time author for childrentopics.com, she has researched various topics in order to provide information to her readers, which expand across 162 countries/territories and every state within the United States. In conducting that research, she discovered that Americans are really struggling in the area of health and wellness, particularly when it comes to proper nutrition, portion control, the need for daily physical exercise, and learning how to dismiss the overabundance of false and misleading information related to all of the above. She decided to make it her mission to educate anyone interested in making a commitment to a lifestyle makeover or modification, and introduced *Get the Real "Skinny" on Healthy Weight Loss*.

I hope that you find the information helpful and that you will see the benefit of learning about the realities of healthy weight loss.

www.randaleeroberts.com

www.ingramcontent.com/pod-product-compliance
Lightning Source LLC
Chambersburg PA
CBHW081653270326
41933CB00017B/3158